Electrical Stimulation and Neuromuscular Disorders

Edited by
W. A. Nix and G. Vrbová

With 56 Figures and 9 Tables

Springer-Verlag
Berlin Heidelberg New York Tokyo

Professor Dr. W. A. Nix
Neurologische Klinik
Universitätskliniken
Langenbeckstr. 1
D-6500 Mainz

Professor Dr. G. Vrbová
Department of Anatomy and
Centre for Neuroscience
University College
Gower Street
London, WC1E 6BT
United Kingdom

ISBN-13: 978-3-642-71339-2 e-ISBN-13: 978-3-642-71337-8
DOI: 10.1007/978-3-642-71337-8

Library of Congress Cataloging-in-Publication Data. Electrical stimulation and neuromuscular disorders. "The papers are the proceedings [of] the First International Symposium on Electrical Stimulation and Neuromuscular Disease in Mainz, West Germany, March 29–30, 1985" – Pref. Includes bibliographies and index. 1. Neuromuscular diseases – Congresses. 2. Electric stimulation – Congresses. I. Nix, W. A. (Wilfred A.), 1947– . II. Vrbová, Gerta. III. International Symposium on Electrical Stimulation and Neuromuscular Disease (1st: 1985: Mainz, Rhineland-Palatinate, Germany) [DNLM: 1. Electrotherapy – congresses. 2. Neuromuscular Diseases – therapy – congresses. WE 550 E38 1985] RC925.5.E44 1986 616.7'40645 86-13052

Softcover reprint of the hardcover 1st edition 1986

2125/3130-543210

Preface

In many cases of neuromuscular disorders the physician is faced with a complete lack of therapeutic approaches. This helplessness places the doctor in a position of conflict between his desire to help and his awareness that there is no treatment. In this situation it is tempting to indiscriminately use any procedure that avoids an admission of medical helplessness while satisfying the patient's demand for treatment. Electrical interventions are often used to avoid this situation. Due to the random use of therapeutic approaches it is not known what really happens.

Presumptions and biased empirical observations have led to the extensive use of different forms of electrical stimulation regimes in neuromuscular diseases. Due to this unsatisfactory situation it is necessary to know more about appropriate methods that are being used in particular disorders.

The search for a better understanding of nerve-muscle interaction has shown that certain activity patterns can influence muscle. These experimental results provide a rational basis for a possible therapeutic use of electrical stimulation of nerve and muscle. Previously most research has been conducted in normal tissue, and little is known regarding the responses of diseased muscle. In an interdisciplinary approach to this, it is our intention to present the current knowledge about basic principles of electrical stimulation in normal muscle. Before electrical stimulation can be accepted as a therapeutic tool, we felt it necessary to summarize the effects of activity in normal and diseased muscle and nerve. Based on animal studies, some stimulation regimes have already been introduced into clinical application. For all of those who wish to know more about the topic, we provide a concise survey of the specific subjects combined with recent findings.

The papers are the proceedings of the First International Symposium on Electrical Stimulation and Neuromuscular Disease in Mainz, West Germany, March 29–30, 1985. We did not attempt to establish any new therapeutic regimens or to achieve a major breakthrough. Rather, the results are meant to show that bringing people together from different disciplines in science and medicine can initiate valuable discussions and serve as a platform to design new experiments.

Mainz/London

WILFRED A. NIX
GERTA VRBOVÁ

Contents

List of Contributors

You will find the addresses at the beginning of the respective contribution

I. Effects of Nerves on Muscle

The Role of Activity in the Development of the Mammalian Motor Unit

G. VRBOVÁ[1]

The Diversity of Motor Units

Mammalian skeletal muscles are usually composed of many motor units, each consisting of a motoneuron and the muscle fibres that the motoneuron supplies. These units are the functional elements that produce movement.

Graded increases of tension are achieved by changing the rate of firing of individual motor units and by recruiting additional units within the same muscle (Adrian and Bronk 1929). Although the variability of firing rate is an important control mechanism in all muscles, there are some muscles, such as the soleus, where the increase in strength is brought about mainly by a recruitment of additional motor units and depends less on frequency modulation (Denny-Brown 1929; Grillner and Udo 1971). This mechanism is known to operate in postural control, while motor units involved in rapid phasic movement show a greater variability of firing rates. Disregarding the differences in frequency coding, there is no doubt that during locomotion the overall activity of postural units exceeds by far that of phasic ones (Freund 1983; Navarrete and Vrbová 1983; Hennig and Lømo 1985). So, for example, the soleus muscle of cats and rabbits, which is composed of postural units, is active no matter whether the animal is standing or walking in its cage, whereas phasic muscles, such as the tibialis anterior or gastrocnemius, are activated only during locomotion. Thus, it is clear that differences between activity patterns of individual motor units do exist. Units active for long periods of time are usually referred to as tonic, whereas those that fire for only brief periods of time are phasic (Vrbová 1963a; Vrbová 1963b; see Freund 1983).

Although these distinctions are to some extent arbitrary, attempts were made to further subdivide phasic units into two groups, according to the readiness at which they are recruited, so that units that are recruited with little effort and produce relatively small forces were said to be different from those that are used only when the muscle is required to produce large forces. Impressed by these differences, Burke and his colleagues classified mammalian motor units into three distinct types, slow fatigue-resistant units (postural), fast fatigue-resistant units (phasic), and fast fatigable units (phasic) (Burke et al. 1973). The classification into these three groups is an oversimplification, for it is known that the excitability of motoneurons and their orderly recruitment forms a functional continuum with no sharp distinctions into three groups (Buchthal and Schmalbruch 1980). This is also reflected in the characteristic properties of muscle fibres, for they, too, vary far more than could be accounted for by a grouping into three types (Pette and Vrbová 1985).

1 Department of Anatomy and Centre for Neuroscience, University College, Gower Street, London WC1E 6BT, U.K.

Electrical Stimulation and Neuromuscular Disorders
Ed. by W. A. Nix and G. Vrbová

The difference in activity patterns of motoneurons is due to their synaptic inputs (Eccles et al. 1957) and their biophysical characteristics, which are determined to some extent by the size of their cell body (Henneman et al. 1965 for review see Freund 1983). In view of this, it is pertinent to mention that the size of motoneurons within a motoneuron pool does not show any grouping, but has a normal distribution (Subramaniam et al. 1985).

Muscle fibres supplied by different types of motoneurons vary with regard to their contractile and biochemical properties (Olson and Swett 1966). Those serving postural motoneurons contract and relax relatively slowly and are classified as type-I fibres according to their histochemical reaction related to differences in the myosin molecule.

The target muscle fibres of phasically active motoneurons are usually fast contracting and relaxing. They are referred to as fast-twitch or type-2 fibres (Burke et al. 1973) that are easily discernible from type-1 fibres because of their strong histochemical reaction for myofibrillar actomyosin adenosine triphosphatase (ATPase).

Postural and phasic motor units also differ in their ability to withstand fatigue: the slow, more active motor units are resistant to fatigue, whereas the intermittently active phasic units can be classified into those that fatigue more readily and those that are less fatiguable. The resistance to fatigue of motor units seems to be correlated to the metabolic properties of the muscle fibres they contain. Muscle fibres of the most fatiguable motor units are characteristically rich in glycolytic enzymes and low in enzymes of aerobic oxidative metabolism. Muscle fibres of fatigue-resistant motor units, no matter whether postural (slow) or phasic (fast), are rich in enzymes of aerobic substrate end-oxidation. Thus, motor units were also classified according to their fatiguability into fast fatiguable (FF), fast fatigue-resistant (FR), and slow fatigue-resistant units (S) (Olson and Swett 1966; Burke et al. 1971; Burke et al. 1973; Kugelberg and Edström 1968; Kugelberg and Lindegren 1979; Németh et al. 1981).

The classification based on fatigability and metabolic properties of the muscle fibres does not necessarily coincide with that based on histochemical reactions for actomyosin ATPase. Nevertheless, in normal adult muscles slow-type-1 fibres are usually oxidative and fatigue resistant (see Pette and Vrbová 1985).

Differences in activity during daily life may account for the large variability of metabolic profiles in different muscle fibres. This may also account for the fact that motor units cannot be rigidly classified into three types, but form a continuum. Circumstantial evidence like this suggests that there is a matching between the metabolic properties of the muscle fibres and the functional characteristics of the motoneuron.

Homogeneity of Individual Motor Units

As opposed to the physiological and biochemical heterogeneity of muscle fibres from a given muscle selected at random, fibres belonging to the same motor unit have nearly identical properties. Using an ingenious method of Kugelberg and Edström (1968) by which muscle fibres from the same motor unit could be 'labelled' by depleting their glycogen by stimulating individual motor axons, it was found that muscle fibres belonging to the same motor unit have a similar histochemical appearance and identical metabolic properties (Nemeth et al. 1981).

The Influence of Innervation on Properties of Muscle

The dependence of the muscle fibre on its neurone was most clearly demonstrated in experiments of Buller et al. (1960b). They sutured the motor nerve from the slow soleus muscle of that cat into the fast flexor digitorum longus and the nerve from this fast muscle into the soleus. Some time after this "cross-innervation", the characteristic contractile speeds of the two muscles were examined and compared with those of the contralateral, unoperated side. The fast muscles now supplied by the slow nerve became slow contracting, and the slow muscles supplied by a fast nerve became fast contracting. By this series of experiments it was clearly established that the contractile properties characteristic of a given muscle are not inherent but are determined by the motor nerve.

It was later found that many other properties characteristic of a slow muscle came to resemble those of a fast muscle when it had become innervated by a nerve from the fast muscle, and vice versa (for review see Pette and Vrbová, 1985).

There are several possible explanations as to how the nerve exerts its influence over the muscle fibres it supplies. In their original paper, Buller et al. (1960b) suggested that the nerve exerts a special "trophic" influence on the muscle fibres and that it is in this way that it determines what is to become of the muscle fibre. Another possible explanation of these results was put forward by A.F. Huxley and discussed by Buller et al. (1960b). Huxley suggested that the motor nerve maintains the slow time course of contraction of the soleus muscle fibres by imposing onto it a slow frequency activity, which may act as a "vibratory stress" (see Buller et al. 1960b). Buller et al. (1960b) did not favour this interpretation, and it was not until later that evidence was provided to show the crucial importance of the activity of the muscle in determining its characteristic properties.

A simple situation was sought that would alter radically the activity pattern of skeletal muscle without interfering with its innervation. Soleus motoneurons have a low threshold to stretch but are not activated by flexor reflex afferens (Eccles et al. 1957). It might therefore be expected that the stretch reflex would be of greater importance for the activity of the soleus than for that of muscles involved in other types of movement. When EMG activity was recorded from the soleus muscles of conscious, unrestrained rabbits, it was found that continuous activity could be recorded from this muscle, no matter whether the rabbit was walking, standing or just sitting quietly in its cage. Other muscles like the tibialis anterior were activated during movement of the animal or on pinching its foot. After cutting the tendons of these muscles, and thus preventing them from being stretched, the continuous activity of soleus motor units can no longer be detected. Tenotomy of the other calf muscles does not alter appreciably their phasic type of EMG activity (Vrbová 1963a).

Thus, tenotomy reduces the activity of the soleus but not that of the tibialis anterior muscle. When the contractile speeds of the tenotomized soleus muscle were examined some time after the operation, it was found that the muscle had become fast contracting. Thus, in this experiment the innervation was unaltered, and only the activity pattern of the soleus muscle was changed by tenotomy, yet the contractile properties of the soleus muscle changed. The activity pattern of the tibialis anterior muscle was unaltered by tenotomy, and correspondingly the contractile speeds remained unaffected (Vrbová 1963b).

In order to study the effects of activity at different frequencies on the contractile properties of muscle, it was thought desirable to work with muscles that had no, or extremely little, reflex activity. The tenotomized soleus, although quiescent, had some activity. If this residual activity was due to a supraspinal excitatory influence on soleus motoneurons, then cutting the spinal cord ought to abolish even this activity. Indeed, after section of the cord the tenotomized muscle is completely "silent", whereas reflex activity can readily be elicited from the tibialis anterior muscle (Vrbová 1963a). The tenotomized soleus of a spinal rabbit became fast contracting, suggesting that its normal activity maintains the slow contractile speed. When the muscles were electrically stimulated at 5 or 10 Hz for 8 h a day over a period of 2 or 3 weeks, the soleus muscle remained slow; when, however, higher frequencies of stimulation were used (20 or 40 Hz) in bursts the soleus muscle became fast contracting. These results clearly show that the contractile speed of the rabbit soleus is determined by the particular activity pattern of the muscle (Vrbová 1966; Salmons and Vrbová 1969).

Whether properties of fast muscles can also be influenced by activity was the next question. Since it is practically impossible to prevent reflex activity from reaching these muscles, it was decided to superimpose a slow 10-Hz-frequency activity onto the normal phasic activity of fast leg muscles. When the contractile characteristics of these stimulated muscles were examined 2–4 weeks after such stimulation, it was found that these fast muscles had become slower contracting. When stimulated for longer intervals such as 2–3 months, their contractile speeds were similar to those of the slow soleus muscle. Thus, even though the slow frequency activity was superimposed onto the normal activity of the muscle, it had a dramatic, slowing effect (Salmons and Vrbová 1969). From these results it is apparent that the nerve exerts its influence on the contractile properties by imposing a particular pattern of activity, and not by a special trophic influence.

Not only the contractile speeds but also the enzyme composition of fast muscles are altered after long-term electrical stimulation. The anaerobic muscle fibres of the tibialis anterior muscle and extensor digitorum longus (EDL) muscles are transformed into predominantly aerobic ones, and this can be shown both by biochemical analysis of the muscles as well as by histochemical examinations (Pette et al. 1973; for review see Pette and Vrbová 1985).

The mechanism by which the muscle fibre alters its biochemical compostion and starts synthesizing a set of different proteins is poorly understood. Experiments where such changes are brought about by electrical stimulation seem to be a suitable model for studying this question.

In adults the contractile properties of muscle fibres are matched almost perfectly to the functional demands of motoneurons that supply them. This is a result of the adaptive changes induced in the muscle by motoneuron activity, and it is because of this that the motor unit can and does function as a true unit, and the muscle fibres are then indeed just an extension of the motoneuron. Yet the muscle fibres are separate individual cells and have no means of intracellular communication with the motoneuron that supplies them. Indeed, during early stages of embryonic development the motoneurons and muscle cells develop independently and do not establish connections with each other until later.

Development of the Matching Properties of Motoneurons and Muscle Fibres

How then does the motor unit develop, and how do the muscle fibres belonging to it acquire those properties that enable them to match the requirement of the motoneurons? It could be that developing muscle cells have special characteristic markers that enable the appropriate motoneuron to recognize and contact them. Muscle cells may, even at these early stages of development, already have an inherent genetic programme that will express specific phenotypic characteristics, recognized by the motoneuron that has contacted them. This hypothesis, while widely accepted among some developmental neurobiologists, (Lance-Jones and Landmesser 1981; Thompson et al. 1984) is very unlikely for the following reasons: (a) during early development even some time after innervation has taken place, the characteristic membrane and contractile properties of all muscle fibres at a comparable stage of development are similar (Gordon et al. 1977); (b) it is relatively easy by surgical manipulations to innervate embryonic muscle by inappropriate nerves (Summerbell and Stirling 1981), and this ability of muscle to accept any alien cholinergic nerve persists in adult animals (Langley and Anderson 1904); and (c) as already mentioned, muscle fibres, embryonic or adult, have an extraordinary capacity to alter their contractile, ultrastructural and biochemical properties (Buller et al. 1960b; Gordon and Vrbová 1975; Ashhurst and Vrbová 1979; Gordon et al. 1981) and are able to alter their phenotype within a wide range in response to changes of activity (Salmons and Vrbová 1969; for review see Pette and Vrbová 1985). Thus, rather than there being a specific recognition during development, it is more likely that the muscle fibres adjust to the particular activity pattern of the motoneuron. That this mechanism operates during development is apparent from results of experiments in which changes of contractile properties and activity patterns with age are simultaneously followed. Although there have been many studies of contractile properties, there is little information as to how they correlate with the activity of the muscle. Close (1964) described the changes of contractile properties of rat soleus (slow) and EDL (fast) muscles during postnatal development. He confirmed that in rats, just like in other mammals (Buller et al. 1960a), both future slow and fast muscles are slowly contracting and relaxing at birth, and with age the contractions of both types of muscles become faster. The increase of speed of contraction continues in EDL, but the contraction of the soleus becomes slower after the initial increase in speed (Close 1964).

Both types of muscles are in rats two to three times slower at birth than 3 weeks later. Moreover, the soleus is unable to maintain tension for long periods of time in response to high-frequency nerve stimulation (Handysides et al. 1986). Thus, the mechanical properties of both muscles are very different from those of adult muscles and would be a poor match for activity patterns generated by motoneurons from older animals. It was therefore of particular interest to establish whether these immature muscles are activated by an activity pattern that matches this early developmental stage.

Evidence is accumulating to show that in newborn animals different classes of motoneurons cannot be distinguished from each other by their particular patterns of activity. Bursian and Sviderskaya (1971) recorded EMG activity from the gastrocnemius muscle of newborn rats and kittens and found that the mean discharge frequency of motor units was low. The adult gastrocnemius is a mixed muscle, composed of different types of motor units. Therefore, these results could mean either that only slow motor units are active at this early stage of development, or that both presumptive slow and fast motor units fire at low rates in neonatal animals. Thus, in order to compare the activity pattern of developing slow and fast units, activity was recorded from muscles with a homogeneous population of motor units; soleus muscles were used for the study of development of slow type motor units and EDL for that of fast motor units (Navarrete and Vrbová 1983).

It has already been stated that in the adult soleus muscle only low-frequency, tonic EMG activity can be recorded. Moreover, even at rest a few motor units maintain regular discharges for several minutes in the absence of any apparent external stimulus. Recruitment of previously silent motor units occurs upon postural activation or during spontaneous locomotion and is accompanied by a very limited increase in the firing rate of the previously active units (Vrbová 1963a; Navarrete and Vrbová 1983; Henning and Lømo 1985).

In newborn rabbits and in rats of up to 12 days of age, the EMG activity of the soleus muscle is strikingly different from the adult. Motor units do not sustain discharges for more than a few seconds, and during spontaneous or reflex activity several motor units are activated synchronously at very low frequencies for a short time. Both postural and nociceptive stimuli produce intermittent activity resembling the phasic pattern of adult fast muscles. At about 12 days of age the soleus muscle undergoes a fundamental change in its pattern of activity. At this time, tonic discharges from single motor units are first detected in the resting animal and during the 3rd week there is a progressive increase in the proportion of tonic motor unit activity and a greater regularity in the discharge of individual motor units. After 3 weeks the basic pattern of activity in the soleus muscle resembles that of the adult (Navarrete and Vrbová 1983). In the EDL of newborn animals the EMG activity is also phasic but unlike in the adult, the firing frequency of the majority of its motor units is relatively low. Although even in the youngest group of animals some motor units reach high instantaneous firing rates during strong activation of the muscle, the vast majority of motor units fire at low frequencies. Thus, during early stages of development both types of motoneurons fire at relatively low rates and are unable to sustain their firing for long periods of time. With development, soleus motoneurons become capable of sustaining their activity for long periods, while motoneurons to EDL start firing at high rates. In addition to these developmental changes in the pattern of activity, there is a several-fold increase in the amount of activity of both types of units during spontaneous movement. Thus, comparing the activity patterns to muscle properties shows that even at this stage there is a matching of muscle properties to motoneuron firing patterns.

Effects of Activity on the Synaptic Organization of the Neuromuscular Junction

If the muscle fibres supplied by a given motoneuron are to match the requirements imposed upon them by this cell, then they can do this best if each muscle fibre is activated only by a single motoneuron. In this case the activity pattern of this motoneuron will be unique to the muscle fibres it innervates.

Indeed, unlike any other excitable cell, mammalian skeletal muscle fibres of adult animals are supplied by only one axon. This situation however is established only after birth, in rats during the first 2 weeks of postnatal development (Redfern 1970). At birth, muscle fibres receive inputs from several motoneurons, but the transition from poly- to mononeuronal innervation is complete almost at the same time as the activity patterns to slow and fast muscles become distinctly different (Brown et al. 1976; O'Brien et al. 1978). The disappearance of polyneuronal innervation and the establishment of the adult pattern of innervation is activity dependent. It fails to take place when nerve activity is reduced (for review see O'Brien et al. 1982) and can be accelerated when nerves to immature muscles are electrically stimulated at low frequencies for only a few hours a day (O'Brien et al. 1978). Thus, the undifferentiated motor-unit activity seen in newborn animals is an essential part of the developmental process that (a) induces the existence of the motor unit in which each muscle fibre is totally committed to a single motoneuron and (b) initiates changes in the muscle cells that enable it to respond to more specialized activity patterns.

Conclusion

Skeletal muscle fibres are unique among excitable cells in that they receive a single neuronal input. An individual motoneuron provides this single input to several muscle fibres so that all of them have an identical activity pattern. In this way the motoneuron and the muscle fibres it supplies form a functional entity, the motor unit.

In adults, the properties of the muscle fibres from the same motor unit are identical and match the requirements of the motoneuron. The matching is brought about by the adaptive change of the muscle fibres in response to the particular activity pattern imposed upon them by the motoneuron. The plasticity of the muscle, i.e. its ability to express particular types of isosymic forms of its contractile and other proteins in response to particular activity patterns, enables the muscle to develop the appropriate phenotype. Therefore, in adults the well-known diversity of motoneuron properties is also reflected by the heterogeneity of muscle fibre types within a muscle, while at the same time muscle fibres belonging to the same motor unit are homogeneous.

It is apparent then that for a precise matching of motoneuron activity and muscle fibre phenotype it is essential that each individual muscle fibre serve only a single motoneuron. While this is the case in adults, in newborn mammals this is not so, and individual muscle fibres are supplied by more than one axon. The transition from polyneuronal to mononeuronal innervation that takes place during development is activity dependent, but the activity patterns of newborn animals that bring about this change are very different from those of adults and match the poorly differentiated physiological properties of the target muscles. The highly specialized activity patterns of adult motoneurons develop later, when each muscle fibre is supplied by a single input and it is then that (a) fully coordinated movement is possible and (b) the diversity of motor units can be established.

Thus, the development of the mammalian motor unit follows this sequence: 1) a poorly specialized activity of motoneurons to muscles of newborn animals brings about the unique situation whereby each muscle fibre is supplied by a single input, and 2) the specialized and differentiated activity patterns of motoneurons in more mature animals, in which the nervous system has become able to produce coordinated movement, induce the phenotypic specialization that leads to the perfect matching of muscle properties to the functional demands of the nervous system.

References

Adrian ED, Bronk DW (1929) The frequency of discharge in reflex and voluntary contraction. J Physiol 67:119–151

Ashhurst ED, Vrbová G (1979) Experimentally induced differentiation of slow tonic and fast twitch muscles of the chick. J Cell Sci 36:137–154

Brown MC, Jansen JKS, Van Essen D (1976) Polyneuronal innervation of individual skeletal muscle fibres in newborn rats and its elimination during maturation. J Physiol 261:387–422

Buchthal F, Schmalburch H (1980) Motor unit of mammalian muscle. Physiol Rev 60:90–142

Buller AJ, Eccles JC, Eccles RM (1960a) Differentiation of fast and slow muscles in the cat hind limb. J Physiol 150:399–416

Buller AJ, Eccles JC, Eccles RM (1960b) Interactions between motoneurones and muscles in respect of the characteristic speeds of their responses. J Physiol 150:417–439

Burke RE, Levine DN, Tsairis P, Engel WK (1971) Mammalian motor units: Physiological-histochemical correlation in three types of motor units in cat gastrocnemius. Science 174:709–712

Burke RE, Levine DN, Tsairis P, Zajac FE (1973) Physiological types and histochemical profiles in motor units of the cat gastrocnemius. J Physiol 234:723–748

Bursian AV, Sviderskaya GE (1971) Studies on the activity of motor units in newborn rats and kittens (in Russian). J Evol Biochem Physiol 7:255–261

Close R (1964) Dynamic properties of fast and slow skeletal muscles of the rat during development. J Physiol 173:74–95

Denny-Brown D (1929) On the nature of postural reflexes. Proc Soc Exp Biol Med 104:252–301

Eccles JC, Eccles RM, Lundberg A (1957) The convergence of monosynaptic excitatory afferents on many different species of alpha motoneurones. J Physiol 142:275–291

Freund HJ (1983) Motor unit and muscle activity in voluntary motor control. Physiol Rev 63:387–436

Gordon T, Vrbová G (1975) The influence of innervation on the differentiation of contractile speeds of developing chick muscles. Pflugers Arch 360:199–218

Gordon T, Purves RD, Vrbová G (1977) Differentiation of electrical and contractile properties of slow and fast muscle fibres. J Physiol 269:535–547

Gordon T, Vrbová G, Willcock G (1981) The influence of innervation on differentiating tonic and twitch muscle fibres of the chicken. J Physiol 319:261–269

Grillner S, Udo M (1971) Recruitment in the tonic stretch reflex. Acta Physiol Scand 81:571–573

Handysides NSP, Navarrete R, O'Brien RAD, Vrbová O (1986) Postnatal changes of slow and fast muscle of the rat (to be published)

Henneman E, Somjen G, Carpenter DO (1965) Functional significance of cell size in spinal motor neurones. J Neurophysiol 28:560–580

Henning R, Lømo T (1985) Firing patterns of motor units in normal rats. Nature 314:164–166

Kugelberg E, Edström L (1968) Differential histochemical effects of muscle contractions on phosphorylase and glycogen in various types of fibres. J Neurol Neurosurg Psychiatry 31:415–423

Kugelberg E, Lindegren B (1979) Transmission and contraction fatigue of rat motor units in relation to succinate dehydrogenese activity of motor unit fibres. J Physiol 288:285–300

Lance-Jones C, Landmesser L (1981) Pathway selection by chick lumbosacral motoneurones during normal development. Proc R Soc Lond [Biol] 214:1–18

Langley JN, Anderson HR (1904) The union of different kinds of nerve fibres. J Physiol 31:365–391

Navarrete R, Vrbová G (1983) Changes of activity patterns in slow and fast muscles during postnatal development. Dev Brain Res 8:11–19

Navarrete R, Vrbová G (1984) Differential effect of nerve injury at birth on the activity pattern of reinnervated slow and fast muscles of the rat. J Physiol 351:675–685

Németh PM, Pette D, Vrbová G (1981) Comparison of enzyme activities among single muscle fibres within defined motor units. J Physiol 311:489–495

O'Brien RAD, Östberg AJC, Vrbová G (1978) Observation on the elimination of polyneuronal innervation in developing mammalian skeletal muscle. J Physiol 282:571–582

O'Brien RAD, Östberg AJC, Vrbová G (1982) The reorganisation of neuromuscular junctions during development in rats. In: Hoffman JF, Giebisch GH (eds) Membranes in growth and development. Liss, New York, pp 247–257

Olson CB, Swett CP (1966) A functional and histochemical characterization of motor units in a heterogeneous muscle (flexor digitorum longus) of the cat. J Comp Neurol 128:475–497

Pette D, Vrbová G (1985) Neural control of phenotypic expression in mammalian muscle fibres. Muscle Nerve 8:676–689

Pette D, Smith ME, Staudte HW, Vrbová G (1973) Effects of long-term electrical stimulation on some contractile and metabolic characteristics of fast rabbit muscles. Pflugers Arch 338:257–272

Redfern P (1970) Neuromuscular transmission in newborn rats. J Physiol 209:701–709

Salmons S, Vrbová G (1969) The influence of activity on some contractile characteristics of mammalian fast and slow muscles. J Physiol 201:535–549

Subramaniam K, Lowrie MB, Vrbová G (1985) The effect of reducing the peripheral field on motoneurone development of the rat. Dev Brain Res 19:11–20

Summerbell D, Stirling RV (1981) The innervation of dorso-ventrally reversed chick wings: evidence that motor axons do not actively seek out their appropriate targets. J Embryol Exp Morphol 61:233–247

Thompson WJ, Sutton J, Riley A (1984) Fibre type composition of single motor units during synapse elimination in neonatal rat soleus muscle. Nature 309:709

Vrbová G (1963a) Changes in motor reflexes produced by tenotomy. J Physiol 166:241–250

Vrbová G (1963b) The effect of motoneurone activity on the speed of contraction of striated muscle. J Physiol 169:513–526

Vrbová G (1966) Factors determining the speed of contraction of striated muscle. J Physiol 185:17–18P

Skeletal Muscle Adaptation in Response to Chronic Stimulation*

D. PETTE[1]

Introduction

Chronic stimulation has become an attractive model for studying activity-induced adaptations and for investigating the role of impulse activity upon phenotype expression in skeletal muscle (for reviews see Jolesz and Sréter 1981; Pette 1984; Pette and Vrbová 1985; Salmons and Henriksson 1981).

The importance of motoneuron activity in the long-term control of mammalian muscles' contractile properties was demonstrated more than 20 years ago by G. Vrbová (Vrbová 1963). She observed that a long-term decrease in impulse activity following tenotomy shortened contraction and relaxation times of rabbit soleus muscle, whereas increases in impulse activity following tenotomy of synergists caused a slowing of contraction in both fast and slow-twitch muscles. Further evidence for the role of impulse activity in determining contractile properties of muscles came from experiments performed a few years later in collaboration with S. Salmons (Salmons and Vrbová 1969). It was then shown that chronic indirect stimulation of rabbit and cat fast-twitch muscles at 10 Hz, a frequency resembling that normally delivered to a slow-twitch muscle, had a pronounced slowing effect on the time courses of both contraction and relaxation. These observations have since been confirmed and extended in many laboratories.

Fast-to-Slow Transitions by Low Frequency Stimulation

Chronic low frequency stimulation of rabbit fast-twitch muscles (e.g., m. tibialis anterior, m. extensor digitorum longus) elicits transformation processes which ultimately turn a "white", fatigable fast-twitch into a "red", less fatigable slow-twitch muscle. This transformation affects the major functional elements of the muscle fiber, i.e., Ca^{2+} regulatory system, energy metabolism, and myofibrillar apparatus. Changes in metabolic enzyme activities, as well as slowing of contraction (time to peak tension), become detectable after brief (48 h) stimulation periods (Heilig and Pette 1980; Heilmann and Pette 1979). Prolonged stimulation progressively increases these changes and finally leads to an apparently complete fast-to-slow transformation (Salmons and Sréter 1976).

* This work was supported by the *Deutsche Forschungsgemeinschaft, Sonderforschungsbereich* 138 *"Biologische Grenzflächen und Spezifität"* and *Sonderforschungsbereich* 156 *"Mechanismen zellulärer Kommunikation"*

1 Faculty of Biology, University of Konstanz, Konstanz, Federal Republic of Germany

Electrical Stimulation and Neuromuscular Disorders
Ed. by W. A. Nix and G. Vrbová

CA^{2+} Regulatory System

Time course studies have revealed an almost twofold increase in time to peak tension during the first 2 weeks of stimulation of a fast-twitch muscle with subsequent increases occurring more slowly. It appears that the early part of this biphasic change results from the altered dynamics of Ca^{2+} release and sequestration, and that the later increases in contraction time are due to an altered myosin composition (Heilmann and Pette 1979). This latter point is supported by the finding that changes in the myosin light chain complement, indicative of a fast-to-slow transition, can be detected electrophoretically only in fast-twitch muscles that are stimulated 24 h daily for more than 3 weeks (Pette et al. 1976; Salmons and Sréter 1976; Sréter et al. 1973). On the other hand, sarcoplasmic reticulum (SR) preparations isolated from 48 h stimulated muscles show significant decreases both in initial rate and maximum capacity of Ca^{2+} uptake (Heilmann and Pette 1979). These changes increase with longer stimulation and are paralleled by decreases in the activity of the Ca^{2+} transport adenosine triphosphatase (ATPase) (Heilmann and Pette 1979; Klug et al. 1983). Electrophoretic analyses indicate that prolonged stimulation of a fast-twitch muscle leads to a type-specific transformation of the SR such that its peptide pattern is indistinguishable from a typically slow-twitch muscle. Similarly, stimulation induces a rearrangement of the phospholipid matrix of the SR membranes (Sarzala et al. 1982).

These functional and biochemical changes of the SR in chronically stimulated fast-twitch muscles correlate well with ultrastructural findings. It has been shown by electron microscopy that the volume densities of T-tubules, terminal cisternae, and longitudinal sarcoplasmic reticulum decrease during chronic low frequency stimulation (Eisenberg and Salmons 1981; Eisenberg et al. 1984). In addition, freeze-fractured SR vesicles reveal a lowered asymmetry of the membrane and a decrease in the 7–9 nm intramembranous particles which are believed to represent the Ca^{2+}-pumping ATPase (Heilmann et al. 1981).

Energy Metabolism

Initial biochemical studies performed on chronically stimulated fast-twitch muscle revealed pronounced effects on activity and isozyme patterns of enzymes in energy metabolism (Pette et al. 1972, 1973). These changes may be summarized as a "white-to-red" transformation and consist mainly of pronounced increases in activity levels of enzymes functioning in the terminal pathways of mitochondrial substrate oxidation (citric acid cycle, fatty acid oxidation, respiratory chain). The increase in these mitochondrial enzymes is pronounced and can be observed qualitatively using appropriate enzyme histochemical markers (Fig. 1).

The changes in the activity pattern of mitochondrial enzymes are accompanied by an increase in myoglobin content (Pette et al. 1973), a rise in capillary density, and a greater functional hyperemia and oxygen consumption during contractile activity (Brown et al. 1976; Hudlická et al. 1977, 1982a). It is probable that these changes, together with the increase in aerobic oxidative capacity, are responsible for the pronounced increase in resistance to fatigue which is a typical effect of chronic stimula-

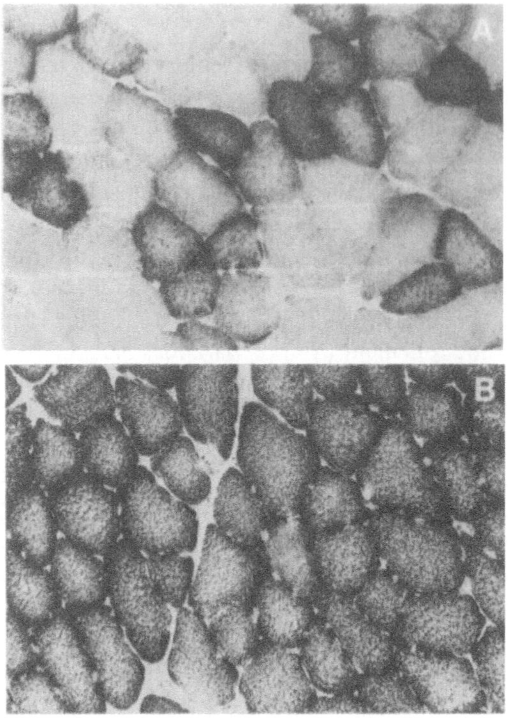

Fig. 1A, B. Histochemical staining for succinate dehydrogenase activity in cross-sections of (**A**) contralateral, unstimulated and of (**B**) 28-day indirectly stimulated (10 Hz, 8 h daily) rabbit tibialis anterior muscles. (From Pette et al. 1973)

tion (Brown et al, 1976; Hudlická et al. 1977; Peckham et al. 1973; Pette et al. 1975; Salmons and Sréter 1976).

The increase in aerobic oxidative capacity is accompanied by a reduction in the potential for anaerobic energy supply. Glycogenolytic and glycolytic enzyme activities decrease (Heilig and Pette 1980; Pette et al. 1972, 1973) and total cellular activity of creatine kinase is likewise reduced (Pette et al. 1973; Schmitt and Pette 1985). However, this decrease in creatine kinase applies only to its cytosolic isozymes, as its mitochondrial isozyme increases markedly and, therefore, follows the rise of enzymes of terminal substrate oxidation (Schmitt and Pette 1985).

The rise in mitochondrial enzyme activities is paralleled by an increase in the fractional volume of mitochondria. A recent chronic stimulation study, combining enzyme activity measurements with electron microscopic morphometry (Reichmann et al. 1985), indicates that the absolute rise in enzymes of the citric acid cycle and of fatty acid oxidation agrees (both in time course and in extent) with the increase in volume density of total mitochondria. However, some mitochondrial enzymes representing special functions, e.g. ketone body utilization or the glycerolphosphate shuttle, appear to change independently (Pette et al. 1973; 1976; Reichmann et al. 1985). Therefore, the mitochondrial population in chronically stimulated fast-twitch muscle differs qualitatively, as well as quantitatively, from that in normal fast-twitch muscle.

Myofibrillar Apparatus

As mentioned above, slowing of contraction results from alterations in Ca^{2+} dynamics and subsequently from a fast-to-slow transformation of the myofibrillar apparatus. Prolonged stimulation induces ultrastructural changes of the Z-bands which widen and finally resemble those in slow-twitch fibers (Eisenberg and Salmons 1981; Eisenberg et al. 1984; Salmons et al. 1978). Histochemical staining for myofibrillar actomyosin ATPase shows a progressive increase in percentage of type I fibers at the cost of type II (Fig. 2). Although the total number of fibers is retained in chronically stimulated fast-twitch muscle (Pette et al. 1976; Salmons and Henriksson 1981), there is a significant drop in weight and cross-sectional area (Fig. 2). The mean size of the muscle fibers decreases and this decrease is due to a reduction in size of the largest fibers (Pette et al. 1975).

Long-term (2–3 months) stimulated fast-twitch muscles appear to be composed entirely of type-I fibers, as judged from histochemical staining for myofibrillar ATPase (Buchegger et al. 1984; Pette 1984). As can be demonstrated by electrophoretic analyses of peptide patterns, the phenotype-specific transformation of myofibrillar proteins is not complete at this time (Buchegger et al. 1984).

Although only selected items have been studied so far, it seems that long-term stimulation leads to a thorough rearrangement of the myofibrillar proteins in the sense of a fast-to-slow transformation of the sarcomere. Changes have been observed for regulatory proteins associated with the thin filament (tropomyosin subunit composition (Roy et al. 1979) and its fast-slow isotypes (Pette 1986), type-I protein

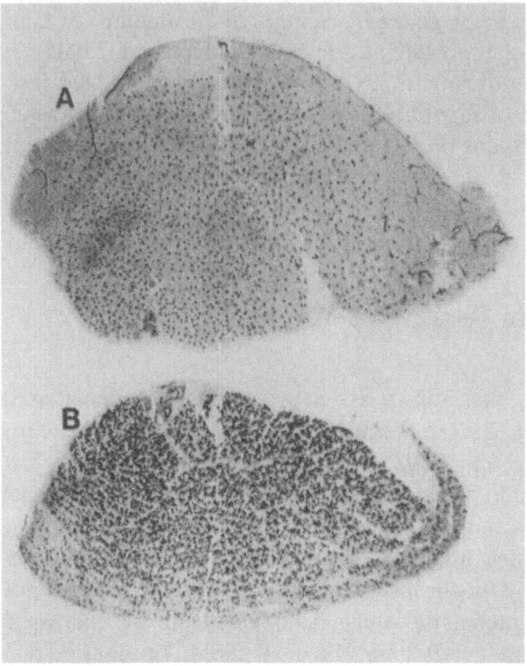

Fig. 2A, B. Histochemical staining for myofibrillar actomyosin ATPase after acid (pH 4.3) preincubation in whole cross-sections of (**A**) contralateral, unstimulated and (**B**) 39-day indirectly stimulated (10 Hz, 24 h daily) rabbit tibialis anterior muscles. Type I fibers stain dark, type II light. (From Pette et al. 1976)

(Heilig et al. 1986; Pette 1986), and protein components of the thick filament. Among these, myosin has been the most extensively studied. Stimulation-induced changes in myosin composition were first detected by alterations in the myosin light chain pattern (Pette et al. 1976; Sréter et al. 1973). Time course studies on the transitions in the light chain pattern reveal that although fast isotypes are symmetrically exchanged with their slow type counterparts, phosphorylatable and alkali light chains follow different time courses (Brown et al. 1983; Seedorf et al. 1983). Stimulation-induced alterations also occur in the heavy chain complement (Brown et al. 1983; Mabuchi et al. 1982; Sréter et al. 1975) and may precede those of the light chains (Brown et al. 1983). It appears, therefore, that the protein components of the myofibrillar apparatus are exchanged asynchronously.

RNA Metabolism

There is increasing evidence that the changes in phenotype expression of chronically stimulated fast-twitch muscle result from altered transcriptional and translational activities. Changes in RNA metabolism are indicated by an almost threefold elevation of total RNA content during the first 2 weeks of stimulation (Pette 1984; Pette et al. 1984; Pluskal and Sréter 1983). This increase is mainly due to the fraction of ribosomal RNA. Indeed, there is a severalfold increase in polysomes reaching a maximum at about 3 weeks of stimulation (Kirschbaum et al. 1985). This change suggests an enhanced translational capacity of stimulated muscle.

Alterations in transcriptional activity have been observed using in vitro translation studies with purified poly(A)RNA preparations. Changes in tissue levels of several proteins (parvalbumin, citrate synthetase, M- and H-subunits of lactate dehydrogenase) have been shown to be preceded by changes in the amounts of their in vitro translatable mRNA (Leberer et al. 1985; Pette 1984; Seedorf et al. 1985). It is clear from the in vitro translation of total mRNA in chronically stimulated fast-twitch muscle that the appearance of myofibrillar proteins specific of slow-twitch fibers e.g., slow-type myosin light chains (Heilig and Pette 1983; Pluskal and Sréter 1983) or "type-I protein" (Heilig et al. 1986), results from translation of newly transcribed mRNA species.

Stimulation-Induced Changes in Denervated Muscle

Transformation processes have also been shown to occur in stimulated, denervated muscle (Lømo et al. 1974, 1980, 1985), as well as in uninnervated myotubes in vitro (Düsterhöft and Pette 1985; Srihari and Pette 1981). It has been shown that low frequency stimulation of denervated soleus muscle of the guinea pig counteracts atrophy of the majority of the fibers and, as judged from qualitative histochemistry, maintains normal levels of enzymes involved in aerobic oxidative metabolism (Nemeth 1982). Similar results have been observed in low frequency stimulated, denervated fast-twitch muscles of the rabbit which do not develop the increased fatigability typical of denervated muscle (Nix 1986; Nix et al. 1985). This may be due to normal or even slightly elevated activity levels of mitochondrial enzymes of terminal substrate oxidation (Reichmann and Nix 1985).

Maintenance and regulation of contractile properties by chronic stimulation of denervated rat muscles have been extensively studied by Lømo and coworkers (Lømo et al. 1974, 1980, 1985). According to these authors, contractile properties of denervated fast and slow-twitch muscles are modified by changes in stimulus pattern. Low-frequency stimulation keeps the denervated soleus muscle slow and turns denervated extensor digitorum longus (EDL) into a slower contracting muscle. Conversely, intermittent high frequency stimulation keeps denervated EDL fast and markedly increases the contraction velocity of denervated soleus. Collaborative biochemical studies on these muscles are currently underway. Preliminary results of enzyme activity determinations, isozyme studies, and analyses of functional proteins of the sarcoplasmic reticulum confirm Lømo's findings and emphasize the specificity of the stimulus pattern for maintenance and transformation of phenotype-specific properties in denervated fast and slow-twitch muscles (T. Lømo, E. Leberer, D. Pette, unpublished observations, 1985). Because neurotrophic factors can be excluded using stimulated, denervated muscle, these findings point to the importance of impulse activity per se and the importance of tonic and phasic impulse patterns in determining expression as well as maintenance of phenotype specific properties.

The question of the specificity of the impulse pattern is less clear in the case of chronically stimulated, innervated muscle. Fast-to-slow transformation using chronic low frequency stimulation of fast-twitch muscle is in agreement with the suggested specificity of the stimulus pattern. However, stimulation of innervated fast-twitch muscles with phasic, high frequency patterns results in apparently similar transformations (Hudlická et al. 1980, 1982b, 1984; Sréter et al. 1982). This apparent discrepancy may be due to inappropriate experimental conditions, i.e., that the applied stimulation protocols may not have mimicked physiologically occurring phasic impulse patterns with regard to frequency and/or average amount of activity typical of fast motor units (Hennig and Lømo 1985). Additionally, it is unknown to what extent the applied stimulus pattern acts directly or elicits reflex motor activity which by itself induces transformation of the muscle (Pette and Vrbová 1985). Further experimentation is needed to clarify this point.

Concluding Remarks

It is apparent that chronic stimulation is capable of determining expression, as well as maintenance of phenotype-specific properties in innervated and denervated fast and slow-twitch muscles. As demonstrated in low-frequency stimulated fast-twitch muscle, transformations appear to result from altered gene expression (primarily alterations in transcription). The main functional elements of the muscle fiber respond in an orderly time sequence (Pette 1984; Pette and Vrbová 1985). Therefore, a fast-twitch, "white" muscle can be turned metabolically "red" by relatively brief stimulation periods without transforming its fast-type myofibrillar apparatus. On the other hand, it is obvious that a fast-twitch muscle which is turned slow by long-term stimulation has a slow-type myofibrillar apparatus and will always be metabolically "red".

These observations indicate that the ultimate fast-to-slow transformation of chronically stimulated fast-twitch muscle results from orderly sequential transitions of the preexisting fiber population. Recent observations indicate that some degenerative/regenerative processes occur initially in chronically stimulated fast-twitch muscle (Maier et al. 1986). However, fiber degeneration apparently involves the fast-glycolytic fiber population. These fibers may not be metabolically prepared to meet sustained contractile activity and may be damaged. They are replaced by newly formed fibers originating from proliferating satellite cells. Although this point needs further experimental study, it should be considered when stimulation is applied to pathological muscle. On the other hand, there is sufficient evidence that chronic stimulation has many beneficial effects, e.g., increased capillarization, enhanced translational activity (protein synthesis), and maintenance of various functional and phenotype-specific properties. To date its application as a possible therapeutic measure involves still unsolved technical problems, such as efficiently stimulating large denervated muscles or muscle groups.

References

Brown MD, Cotter MA, Hudlická O, Vrbová G (1976) The effects of different patterns of muscle activity on capillary density, mechanical properties and structure of slow and fast rabbit muscles. Pflügers Arch 361:241–250

Brown WE, Salmons S, Whalen RG (1983) The sequential replacement of myosin subunit isoforms during muscle type transformation induced by long term electrical stimulation. J Biol Chem 258:14686–14692

Buchegger A, Nemeth PM, Pette D, Reichmann H (1984) Effects of chronic stimulation on the metabolic heterogeneity of the fibre population in rabbit tibialis anterior muscle. J Physiol (Lond) 350:109–119

Düsterhöft S, Pette D (1985) Changes in myosin light chains by chronic stimulation of chick myotubes in culture. J Physiol (Lond) 361:33P

Eisenberg BR, Salmons S (1981) The reorganization of subcellular structure in muscle undergoing fast-to-slow type transformation. Cell Tissue Res 220:449–471

Eisenberg BR, Brown JMC, Salmons S (1984) Restoration of fast muscle characteristics following cessation of chronic stimulation. Cell Tissue Res 238:221–230

Heilig A, Pette D (1980) Changes induced in the enzyme activity pattern by electrical stimulation of fast-twitch muscle. In: Pette D (ed) Plasticity of muscle. de Gruyter, Berlin, pp 409–420

Heilig A, Pette D (1983) Changes in transcriptional activity of chronically stimulated fast twitch muscle. FEBS Lett 151:211–214

Heilig A, Seedorf U, Pette D (1986) Appearance of type-I-protein and its mRNA in rabbit fast-twitch muscle as induced by chronic stimulation. J Muscle Res Cell Motil 7:59

Heilmann C, Pette D (1979) Molecular transformations in sarcoplasmic reticulum of fast-twitch muscle by electro-stimulation. Eur J Biochem 93:437–446

Heilmann C, Müller W, Pette D (1981) Correlation between ultrastructural and functional changes in sarcoplasmic reticulum during chronic stimulation of fast muscle. J Membr Biol 59:143–149

Hennig R, Lømo T (1985) Firing patterns of motor units in normal rats. Nature (Lond) 314:164–166

Hudlická O, Brown M, Cotter M, Smith M, Vrbová G (1977) The effect of long-term stimulation of fast muscles on their blood flow, metabolism and ability to withstand fatigue. Pflügers Arch 369:141–149

Hudlická O, Tyler KR, Aitman T (1980) The effect of long-term electrical stimulation on fuel uptake and performance in fast skeletal muscles. In: Pette D (ed) Plasticity of muscle. de Gruyter, Berlin, pp 401–408

Hudlická O, Dodd L, Renkin EM, Gray SD (1982a) Early changes in fiber profile and capillary density in long-term stimulated muscles. Am J Physiol 243:H528–H535

Hudlická O, Tyler KR, Srihari T, Heilig A, Pette D (1982b) The effect of different patterns of long-term stimulation on contractile properties and myosin light chains in rabbit fast muscles. Pflügers Arch 393:164–170

Hudlická O, Aitman T, Heilig A, Leberer E, Tyler KR, Pette D (1984) Effects of different patterns of long-term stimulation on blood flow, fuel uptake and enzyme activities in rabbit fast skeletal muscles. Pflügers Arch 402:306–311

Jolesz F, Sréter FA (1981) Development, innervation, and activity pattern induced changes in skeletal muscle. Ann Rev Physiol 43:531–552

Kirschbaum BJ, Seedorf U, Pette D (1986) Changes of the translational apparatus in chronically stimulated rabbit fast-twitch muscle. J Muscle Res Cell Motil 7:60

Klug G, Wiehrer W, Reichmann H, Leberer E, Pette D (1983) Relationships between early alterations in parvalbumins, sarcoplasmic reticulum and metabolic enzymes in chronically stimulated fast twitch muscle. Pflügers Arch 399:280–284

Leberer E, Seedorf U, Klug G, Pette D (1985) Parvalbumin levels and in vitro translation of its mRNA in chronically stimulated rabbit muscle. J Muscle Res Cell Motil 6:84

Lømo T, Westgaard RH, Dahl HA (1974) Contractile properties of muscle: control by pattern of muscle activity in the rat. Proc R Soc Lond [Biol] 187:99–103

Lømo T, Westgaard RH, Engebretsen L (1980) Different stimulation patterns affect contractile properties of denervated rat soleus muscles. In: Pette D (ed) Plasticity of muscle. de Gruyter, Berlin, pp 297–309

Lømo T, Gundersen K, Hennig R, Westgaard R (1985) The role of impulse patterns in maintaining and regulating contractile properties in intact and chronically denervated and stimulated rat skeletal muscles. In: Eccles JC, Dimitrijevic MR (eds) Recent achievements in restorative neurology. 1 Upper motor neuron functions and dysfunctions. Karger, Basel, pp 249–262

Mabuchi K, Szvetko D, Pintér K, Sréter FA (1982) Type IIB to IIA fiber transformation in intermittently stimulated rabbit muscles. Am J Physiol 242:C373–C381

Maier A, Gambke B, Pette D (1986) Degeneration-regeneration as a mechanism contributing to the fast to slow conversion of chronically stimulated fast-twitch muscle. Cell Tissue Res 244: 635–643

Nemeth PM (1982) Electrical stimulation of denervated muscle prevents decreases in oxidative enzymes. Muscle Nerve 5:134–139

Nix WA (1986) Maintenance of muscle integrity. In: Dimitrijevic M, Kakulas BA, Vrbová G (eds) Recent achievements in restorative neurology, vol 2. Karger, Basel, pp 332–340

Nix WA, Reichmann H, Schröder JM (1985) Influence of direct low frequency stimulation on contractile properties of denervated fast-twitch muscle of the rabbit. Pflügers Arch 405:244–249

Peckham PH, Mortimer JT, von der Meulen JP (1973) Physiologic and metabolic changes in white muscle of cat following induced exercise. Brain Res 50:424–429

Pette D (1984) Activity-induced fast to slow transitions in mammalian muscle. Med Sci Sports Exerc 16:517–528

Pette D (1986) Motoneurone activity and phenotype expression of muscle fibers. In: Dimitrijevic M, Kakulas BA, Vrbová G (eds) Recent achievements in restorative neurology, vol 2. Karger, Basel, pp 265–275

Pette D, Vrbová G (1985) Invited review: Neural control of phenotype expression in mammalian muscle fibers. Muscle Nerve 8:676–689

Pette D, Staudte HW, Vrbová G (1972) Physiological and biochemical changes induced by long-term stimulation of fast muscle. Naturwissenschaften 59:469–470

Pette D, Smith ME, Staudte HW, Vrbová G (1973) Effects of long-term electrical stimulation on some contractile and metabolic characteristics of fast rabbit muscles. Pflügers Arch 338:257–272

Pette D, Ramirez BU, Müller W, Simon R, Exner GU, Hildebrand R (1975) Influence of intermittent long-term stimulation on contractile, histochemical and metabolic properties of fibre populations in fast and slow rabbit muscles. Pflügers Arch 361:1–7

Pette D, Müller W, Leisner E, Vrbová G (1976) Time dependent effects on contractile properties, fibre population, myosin light chains and enzymes of energy metabolism in intermittently and continuously stimulated fast twitch muscles of the rabbit. Pflügers Arch 364:103–112

Pette D, Heilig A, Klug G, Reichmann H, Seedorf U, Wiehrer W (1984) Alterations in phenotype expression of muscle by chronic nerve stimulation. In: Strohman RC, Wolf S (eds) Gene expression in muscle. Plenum, New York, pp 169–178

Pluskal MG, Sréter FA (1983) Correlation between protein phenotype and gene expression in adult rabbit fast twitch muscles undergoing a fast to slow fiber transformation in response to electrical stimulation in vivo. Biochem Biophys Res Commun 113:325–331

Reichmann H, Nix WA (1985) Changes of energy metabolism, myosin light chain composition, lactate dehydrogenase isozyme pattern and fibre type distribution of denervated fast-twitch muscle from rabbit after low frequency stimulation. Pflügers Arch 405:244–249

Reichmann H, Hoppeler H, Mathieu-Costello O, von Bergen F, Pette D (1985) Biochemical and ultrastructural changes of skeletal muscle mitochondria after chronic electrical stimulation in rabbits. Pflügers Arch 404:1–9

Roy RK, Mabuchi K, Sarkar S, Mis C, Sréter FA (1979) Changes in tropomyosin subunit pattern in chronic electrically stimulated rabbit fast muscles. Biochem Biophys Res Commun 89:181–187

Salmons S, Henriksson J (1981) The adaptive response of skeletal muscle to increased use. Muscle Nerve 4:94–105

Salmons S, Sréter FA (1976) Significance of impulse activity in the transformation of skeletal muscle type. Nature (Lond) 263:30–34

Salmons S, Vrbová G (1969) The influence of activity on some contractile characteristics of mammalian fast and slow muscles. J Physiol (Lond) 210:535–549

Salmons S, Gale DR, Sréter FA (1978) Ultrastructural aspects of the transformation of muscle fibre type by long term stimulation: changes in Z discs and mitochondria. J Anat 127:17–31

Sarzala MG, Szymanska G, Wiehrer W, Pette D (1982) Effects of chronic stimulation at low frequency on the lipid phase of sarcoplasmic reticulum in rabbit fast-twitch muscle. Eur J Biochem 123:241–245

Schmitt T, Pette D (1985) Increased mitochondrial creatine kinase in chronically stimulated fast-twitch rabbit muscle. FEBS Lett 188:341–344

Seedorf K, Seedorf U, Pette D (1983) Coordinate expression of alkali and DTNB myosin light chains during transformation of rabbit fast muscle by chronic stimulation. FEBS Lett 158:321–324

Seedorf U, Leberer E, Pette D (1985) In vitro translation of mRNAs coding for citrate synthetase and lactate dehydrogenase isozyme 5 in chronically stimulated rabbit muscle. J Muscle Res Cell Motil 6:85–86

Sréter FA, Gergely J, Salmons S, Romanul FCA (1973) Synthesis by fast muscle of myosin characteristic of slow muscle in response to long term stimulation. Nature New Biol (Lond) 241:17–19

Sréter FA, Elzinga M, Mabuchi K, Salmons S, Luff AR (1975) The *N*-methylhistidine content of myosin in stimulated and cross-reinnervated skeletal muscles of the rabbit. FEBS Lett 57:107–111

Sréter FA, Pinter K, Jolesz F, Mabuchi K (1982) Fast to slow transformation of fast muscles in response to long-term phasic stimulation. Exp Neurol 75:95–102

Srihari T, Pette D (1981) Myosin light chains in normal and electrostimulated cultures of embryonic chicken breast muscle. FEBS Lett 123:312–314

Vrbová G (1963) The effect of motoneurone activity on the speed of contraction of striated muscle. J Physiol (Lond) 169:513–526

The Effect of Long-Term Electrical Stimulation on Capillary Supply and Metabolism in Fast Skeletal Muscle

O. Hudlická[1], M. A. Cotter[2], and J. Cooper[3]

Introduction

Salmons and Vrbová (1969) showed that chronic stimulation of rabbit fast muscles at a frequency naturally occurring in nerves to slow muscles (10 Hz continuously) changed the contractile properties towards those characteristic of slow muscles. Subsequent series of experiments (Pette et al. 1973, 1975, 1976, see Pette and Vrbová, 1985) demonstrated the effect of such stimulation on the transformation of the metabolic pattern with an increase in the activity of oxidative and decrease in glycolytic enzymes. It has been known for a long time (Ranvier 1874) that muscles with a high aerobic metabolism have a much better capillary supply than muscles with high glycolytic metabolism. Romanul (1965) showed a higher number of capillaries surrounding fibres with a high activity of oxidative enzymes in one muscle, and Gray and Renkin (1978) found, using quantitative evaluation, twice as many capillaries in relation to fibres with a high activity of succinate dehydrogenase (SDH) than in those with a low SDH activity. Hudlická (1982) showed a very good relationship between the activity of citrate synthase – estimated in many different muscles by Bass et al. (1969) – and capillary density (CD), and Hoppeler et al. (1981) demonstrated significant correlations between the volume density of mitochondria and CD in twenty different muscles of various mammals. It was thus not surprising to find increased capillary supply in chronically stimulated muscles (Cotter et al. 1973). The purpose of this presentation is to summarise the data on the effect of different patterns of long-term electrical stimulation on capillary growth in various muscles of different species, to show the relationship between increased capillary supply, changes in the proportion of oxidative and glycolytic fibres and muscle metabolism and to discuss the importance of increased capillarisation for muscle performance.

The Effect of Different Patterns of Stimulation on Capillary Growth

The low-frequency continuous stimulation, applied for 8 h/day, induced increased capillarisation – demonstrated here mainly as changes in the capillary: fibre (C:F) ratio – in many different muscles in several species (Table 1). The increase in C:F ratio does not seem to be dependent on the initial composition of muscle fibres, as it was much higher in the medial head of rabbit gastrocnemius (by 133%) than in rabbit

1 Department of Physiology, University of Birmingham, Birmingham B15 2TJ, U.K.
2 Department of Physiology, Marischal College, University of Aberdeen, Scotland
3 Department of Surgery, St. George's Medical School, London, U.K.

Electrical Stimulation and Neuromuscular Disorders
Ed. by W. A. Nix and G. Vrbová

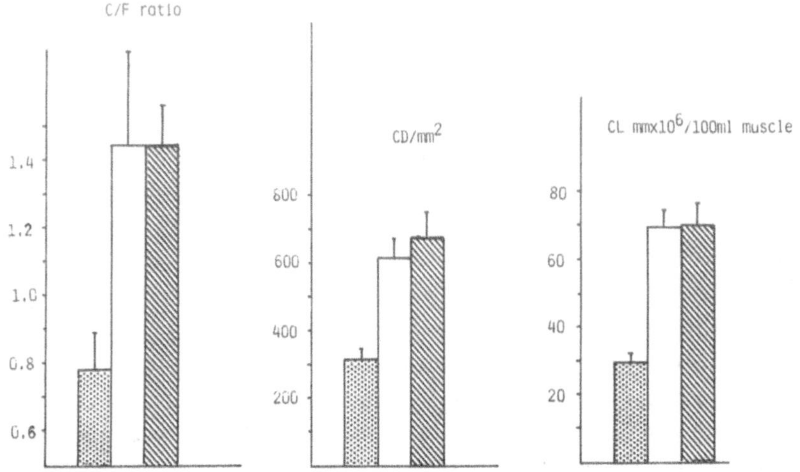

Fig. 1. Capillary supply in different cat muscles: control gracilis ▨, gracilis stimulated for 14–28 days at 10 Hz ■, and soleus □. Data from electron micrographs. Capillary length was estimated from capillary density and a correction factor for tortuosity (according to Mathieu et al. 1983). Data from Hoppeler et al. (1983)

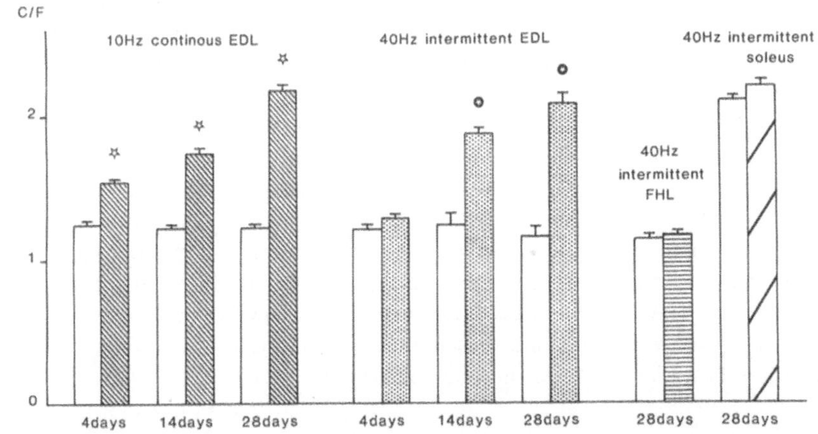

Fig. 2. Capillary : fibre ratios (mean ± S.E.) in different rabbit muscles, stimulated for 8 h/day at various patterns of frequencies. 10 Hz continuous, giving 36000 impulses/h ■. 40 Hz intermittent, 3 trains of 5-s duration each, giving 36000 impulses/h ▨. 40 Hz intermittent, trains of 5-s duration every 100 s, giving 1440 impulses/h ▤ and ▧. □, control; EDL, extensor digitorum longus; FHL, flexor hallucis longus; ☆, $P<0.01$; ●, $P<0.001$. Reproduced from Hudlická (1985) by permission of J Exp Biol

extensor digitorum longus (EDL; by 43%) stimulated for 14 days, although the proportion of glycolytic fibres in these two muscles is not much different (38.9% in gastrocnemius, 43.7% in EDL). Within 14–28 days capillary supply – estimated on the basis of C : F ratio, CD (number of capillaries/mm^2) or capillary length – reached values found in slow muscles (Fig. 1). Myrhage and Hudlická (1978) showed, observ-

Table 1. C:F ratio in different chronically stimulated muscles in various animals. Means ± SE, % of fast glycolytic, fast oxidative and slow fibres in parenthesis, 10-Hz continuous stimulation. 40-Hz trains (5 s on, 3 x/min). *C*, control; *S*, stimulated muscle; *EDL*, extensor digitorum longus, *TA*, tibialis anterior; *EHP*, extensor hallucis proprius

Rabbit	EDL (43.7–51.0–5.3)[c]		TA (39.0–58.0–4.0)[c]		Gastro med. (38.9–37.8–23.2)[b]		Gastro lat. (51.1–34.4–14.5)[b]	
10 Hz	C	S	C	S	C	S	C	S
14 days	1.22 ± 0.02[f]	1.74 ± 0.03*[f]	–	–	1.26 ± 0.09	2.94 ± 0.21*	1.20 ± 0.06	2.74 ± 0.21
28 days		2.18 ± 0.03*[f]	–	–	–	–	–	–
40 Hz								
14 days	1.25 ± 0.02[g]	1.86 ± 0.04*[g]	1.40 ± 0.03[g]	1.83 ± 0.07*[g]				
28 days		2.07 ± 0.06*	–	–				
Rat	EDL (38–59–3)[a]		TA (32–66–2)[a]		EHP (60–25–15)[d]			
10 Hz	C	S	C	S	C	S		
7 days	1.11 ± 0.05	1.31 ± 0.03*	1.35	1.56*	0.99 ± 0.01	1.22 ± 0.04*[e]		
12–14 days						1.36 ± 0.02*		
40 Hz								
7 days	1.15 ± 0.02	1.10 ± 0.025						
Cat	Gracilis (72–13–15)[a]							
10 Hz	C	S						
14–28 days	0.78 ± 0.09	1.45 ± 0.11*[h]						

* Values significantly different from controls
[a] Data from Ariano et al. (1973)
[b] Data from Gray and Renkin (1978)
[c] Data from Hudlická et al. (1982a)
[d] Data from Myrhage and Hudlická (1976)
[e] Data from Myrhage and Hudlická (1978)
[f] Data from Brown et al. (1976)
[g] Data from Hudlická and Tyler (1984)
[h] Data from Hoppeler et al. (1983)

ing microcirculation in rabbit tenuissimus and rat extensor hallucis proprius (EHP) in vivo, that the increase in C:F ratio was due to growth of new capillaries: capillary sprouts started to grow from the bends of preexisting capillaries, gradually connecting as very narrow channels without flow to other capillaries. Flow was established later and the total capillary surface area available for exchange with extravascular space was considerably increased, with a resulting increase in total blood flow at rest (Hudlická and el Khelly 1985) and particularly during contractions (Hudlická et al. 1977, 1984).

In contrast, intermittent tetanic stimulation (trains at 40 Hz 5-s duration every 100 s) did not induce any change in capillary supply either in a fast (flexor hallucis longus) or slow (soleus) muscle (Brown et al. 1976) (Fig. 2). When the total number of impulses was, however, increased to match that used with continuous stimulation at 10 Hz (i.e. 36000/h) by increasing the frequency of trains to 3/min, C:F ratio increased in muscles stimulated for 14 or 28 days to a similar level with both types of stimulation (Table 1, Fig. 2). Both types of stimulation also induced similar changes in contractile properties and myosin light chains (Hudlická et al. 1982b) and muscle metabolism (Hudlická et al. 1984), when applied for a long enough period (14–28 days).

Early Changes in Capillarisation and Muscle Fibre Composition with Different Types of Stimulation

The changes occurring within the first few days of chronic stimulation are dissimilar with different patterns of stimulation and in different muscles. Pette and Tyler (1983) showed a 50% increase in the activity of succinate dehydrogenase (SDH) in IIb fibres in rabbit tibialis anterior after only 4 days of stimulation with 10 Hz; stimulation at 40 Hz produced only a 30% increase in muscles stimulated for 7 days. These quantitative findings support histochemical analysis based on staining for myosin adenosine triphosphatase (ATPase) (Brooke and Kaiser 1969) and SDH (Pearse 1968), which enabled us to find the proportion of fast glycolytic (FG or αW), fast oxidative (FO or αR) and slow oxidative (SO or βR) fibres. As some fast fibres are only faintly stained for SDH, Gray and Renkin (1978) introduced an "intermediate" group (FI or α?). This classification was used to find out changes in fibre composition in rabbit extensor digitorum longus (EDL) and tibialis anterior (TA) stimulated at 10 Hz (Hudlická et al. 1982a) or 40 Hz (Hudlická and Tyler 1984) for 2, 4 and 7 days. Tibialis anterior showed a significant decrease in the proportion of FG and increased proportion of FO fibres after only 2 days of stimulation at 10 Hz, with similarly changed composition in muscles stimulated for 4 days. Stimulation at 40 Hz was without effect on the fibre composition after 4 days, and a decrease in the proportion of glycolytic with an increased proportion of oxidative fibres (mainly FI and SO) only occurred in muscles stimulated for 7 days (Table 2). In contrast, 10 Hz stimulation for 2 or 4 days was without any effect on fibre composition in EDL, and stimulation at 40 Hz produced a significant decrease in the proportion of glycolytic and increase in the proportion of oxidative fibres already after 4 days (Table 2).

Table 2. Proportion (%) of fast glycolytic (αW), fast intermediate (α?), fast oxidative (αR) and slow oxidative (βR) fibres in rabbit tibialis anterior *(TA)* and extensor digitorum longus *(EDL)* stimulated for 2, 4 or 7 days, 8 h/day either continuously at 10 Hz or with trains at 40 Hz (5 s duration 3 x/min). Means ± SEM

	TA							
	10 Hz				40 Hz			
	2 days		4 days		4 days		7 days	
	C	S	C	S	C	S	C	S
αW	37.0 ±1.64	32.0* ±1.27	39.0 ±1.28	32.13* 1.23	36.7 ±1.9	35.6 ±3	41.0 ±1.7	34.2* ±2.4
α?	6.23 ±0.44	7.0 ±1.27	7.47 ±0.44	6.85 0.38	16.3 ±0.9	13.2 ±0.8	11.2 ±1.0	14.9* ±1.1
αR	52.0 ±1.32	56.5* ±1.12	49.52 ±1.02	56.2* 1.20	44.3 ±2.2	48.5 ±2.5	46.2 ±1.5	47.2 ±1.7
βR	4.82 ±0.55	4.49 ±0.37	4.02 ±0.38	4.82 4.02	2.7 ±0.7	2.7 ±0.8	2.2 ±0	3.6* ±0.3
	EDL							
	2 days		4 days		4 days		7 days	
	C	S	C	S	C	S	C	S
αW	44.83 ±1.36	44.89 ±0.9	43.67 ±1.07	43.94 ±0.95	41.9 ±1.8	32.0* ±1.9	40.4 ±1.4	40.8 ±0.9
α?	6.19 ±0.56	8.58 ±0.40	7.48 ±0.55	6.98 ±0.69	15.9 ±0.6	19.8 ±3	13.8 ±0.8	13.8 ±1.5
αR	41.42 ±1.04	41.5 ±1.47	43.56 ±1.10	44.2 ±1.09	37.6 ±1.4	41.2 ±3.9	42.5 ±1.1	37.8* ±0.9
βR	7.56 ±0.249	5.04 ±0.249	5.27 ±0.28	4.94 ±0.38	4.5 ±0.7	5.8 ±1.1	3.6 ±0.5	7.6* ±1.1

* Values significantly different from controls

Growth of capillaries also appeared at different times with the two patterns of stimulation in these two muscles. Capillary density or C:F ratio was not changed in TA stimulated at 10 Hz during the first 4 days or at 40 Hz during the first 7 days (Hudlická et al. 1982a; Hudlická and Tyler 1984). EDL muscles stimulated at 10 Hz for 4 days had a significantly higher C:F ratio (1.54 ± 0.02 compared to 1.25 ± 0.02 in control muscles) but stimulation at 40 Hz was without effect on C:F or CD. Prolongation of this type of stimulation for 7 days resulted in a significant increase in C:F (1.58 ± 0.04) and CD (269 ± 8 cappilaries mm^2) compared with 251 ± 3 in controls. Thus, stimulation at 10 Hz induced growth of capillaries in EDL appearing before the changes in muscle fibre composition, while in TA increased proportion of oxidative fibres preceded the appearance of capillary growth. Stimulation at 40 Hz induced metabolic changes in both muscles before capillary growth was observed.

Why the two muscles show slightly different changes in response to long-term stimulation is open for speculation: rabbit TA has a slightly lower proportion of glycolytic fibres than EDL, and it is possible that the increased metabolic demands during the increased activity could be met in the first place by increased blood supply to the oxidative fibres with their already high capillary supply and the possibility of higher oxygen extraction. On the other hand, this increased activity could produce local hypoxia in EDL which has a higher proportion of glycolytic fibres not adapted to long-lasting contractions. When the distribution of capillaries was analysed with respect to different fibre types, using the method described by Gray and Renkin (1978), it was obvious that the increase in capillary: fibre ratio occurred with both types of stimulation in the vicinity of fibres with a relatively low activity of SDH (Hudlická and Tyler 1984, Fig. 3). This finding would seem to corroborate the assumption that local hypoxia might be an important factor stimulating capillary growth. It was considered in muscles stimulated at 10 Hz (Hudlická and Schroeder 1978; Hudlická et al. 1982a), but its participation seems to be more doubtful in muscles stimulated at 40 Hz: Kanabus et al. (1980) found higher PO_2 in rabbit TA stimulated at 40 Hz for 4 or 7 days at rest with no difference after isometric contractions.

Another possible explanation for capillary growth in chronically stimulated muscles is related to the increase in blood flow, and mechanical factors, such as wall stress (Thoma 1911; Waxman 1981), movements of red blood cells (RBC) (Brånemark 1965) or pressure. The pattern of flow is different with the two types of stimulation: 10-Hz continuous contractions lead to a long-lasting increase, intermittent 40-Hz stimulation not only causes a short period without blood flow at the peak of each tetanus, but the total increase in blood flow per minute is not well main-

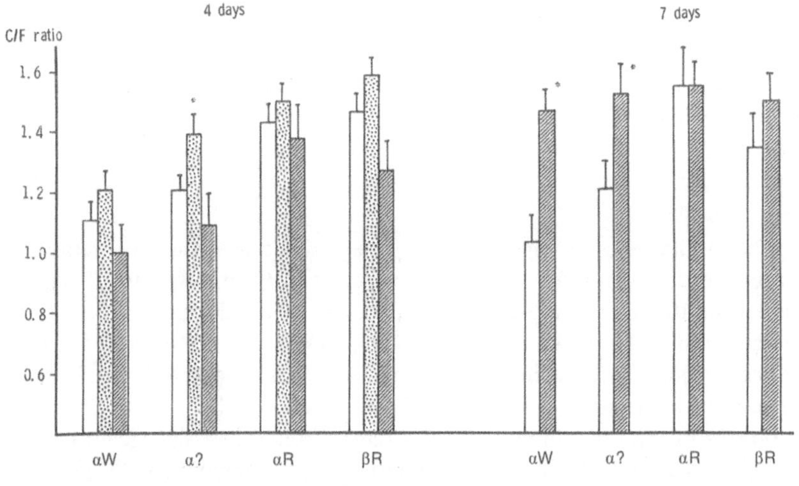

Fig. 3. Rabbit EDL. Capillary: fibre ratio with respect to different fibre types in muscles stimulated continuously at 10 Hz for 4 days, and in muscles stimulated intermittently at 40 Hz for 4 and 7 days. *αW*, fast glycolytic fibres; *αR*, fast oxidative fibres; *α?*, fast fibres on the borderline between glycolytic and oxidative; *βR*, slow oxidative fibres. *Asterisks* denote values significantly different from controls at $P < 0.05$ level. □, control; ▨, stimulated at 10 Hz; ▩, stimulated at 40 Hz. From Hudlická and Tyler (1984) by permission of J Physiol (Lond)

tained over a long period of isotonic contractions during the first hours of stimulation (Aitman et al. 1979).

The increased capillarisation around predominantly glycolytic fibres could only be explained by changes in blood flow if there is a greater increase in flow during muscle contractions in capillaries supplying glycolytic rather than oxidative fibres. The outer three to four layers of rat TA muscle are composed predominantly of glycolytic fibres, while rat soleus is composed almost exclusively of oxidative fibres. When velocity of RBC was studied in capillaries supplying these two muscles, it was found that its increase was greater and more consistent in the former than in the latter (Dawson et al. 1983).

Relationship Between the Increased Capillarisation, Muscle Metabolism and Performance

It is well known that highly oxidative muscles with a dense capillary network do not fatigue, and increased resistance to fatigue was found in rabbit muscles stimulated for 14 or 28 days both at 10 Hz (Pette et al. 1975; Hudlická et al. 1977) and at 40 Hz (Hudlická et al. 1982b). At this stage all stimulated muscles showed already a considerable increase in the activity of oxidative enzymes (Hudlická et al. 1984), as well as increased capillary supply, and it is difficult to decide what is more important for the maintenance of tension. Increased resistance to fatigue was also observed in rabbit muscles stimulated at 10 Hz for only 4 days (Hudlická et al. 1977) when the activity of oxidative enzymes in EDL was not increased (Pette et al. 1973) but C:F ratio was (Brown et al. 1976). In rats, stimulation at 40 Hz caused increased staining for SDH with no change in C:F ratio, while stimulation at 10 Hz did not affect SDH activity and increased C:F ratio (Table 1). It is possible that greater capillary density and surface area enhances the diffusion of oxygen and ensures its more homogeneous supply to different muscle fibres, and hence a more rapid rephosphorylation of ATP and CP. If so it would be expected that chronically stimulated fast muscles would fatigue less only in vivo, with intact blood supply, but not if blood supply were occluded or if the muscles contracted in vitro where the benefit of the increased capillary surface area could not be utilised. Also, the decrease in the content of ATP and CP in such muscles contracting in vivo should be smaller than in control muscles, but hardly any difference should be seen between chronically stimulated and control muscles contracting in vitro. Experiments to test this hypothesis were performed on rat EDL muscle contracting for 5 min at 4 Hz.

It is obvious from Fig. 4 that muscles contracting at 10 Hz fatigued less than the control ones, but the difference disappeared when the femoral artery was occluded immediately before the onset of contractions. The peak tension developed by some stimulated muscles was higher, but the difference was not significant when all muscles were compared (Fig. 5). The tension at the end of the period of contraction expressed as a percentage of the initial tension decreased to $63.5 \pm 7.6\%$ in control (15 muscles) and increased to $104.0 \pm 8.4\%$ in chronically stimulated muscles (9 experiments) ($P < 0.001$). After the occlusion of both femoral arteries 5 min of isometric contractions produced a dramatic decrease in isometric twitch tension in both mus-

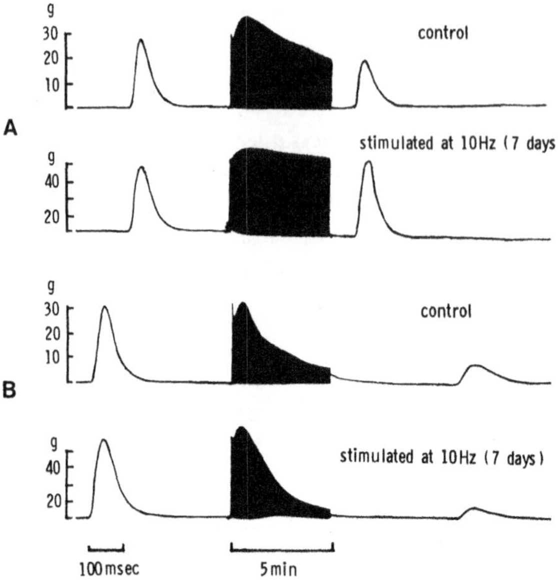

Fig. 4A, B. Record of isometric tension from a control and chronically stimulated rat EDL muscle (10 Hz) in vivo with normal blood supply (**A**) and with tied femoral arteries (**B**)

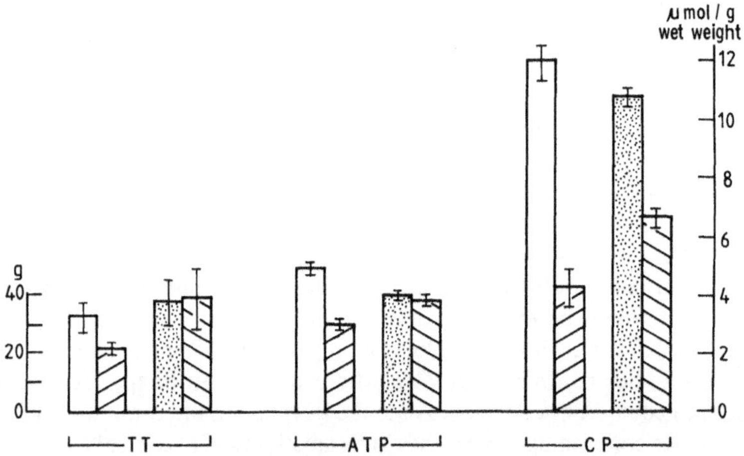

Fig. 5. Twitch tension (in g) and content of ATP and CP (in μmol/g wet weight) in control and chronically stimulated rat EDL muscles at rest and at the end of 5-min isometric contractions (at 4 Hz) in vivo. □, control muscles at rest; ▨, control muscles contracting; ▩, chronically stimulated muscles at rest; ▧, chronically stimulated muscles contracting

cles (Fig. 4) to 22.1 ± 1.6% in control and 17.4 ± 3.0% in chronically stimulated ones.

The content of ATP after 5 min of contractions was significantly lower in control muscles (4.88 ± 0.13 μmol/g wet weight as opposed to 2.7 ± 0.25 μmol/g wet weight, $P < 0.001$) and did not show any difference in chronically stimulated muscles, although the initial levels were lower – similar to lower levels found in slow muscles

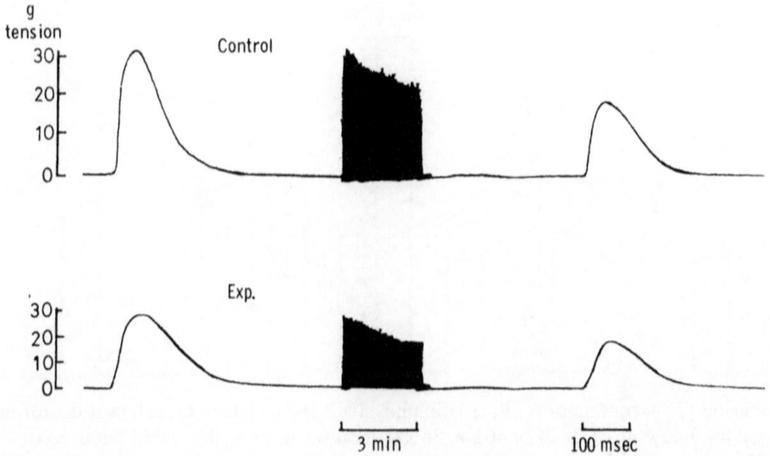

Fig. 6. Record of isometric tension from a control (*upper part*) and chronically stimulated (10 Hz) (*lower part*) rat EDL in vitro

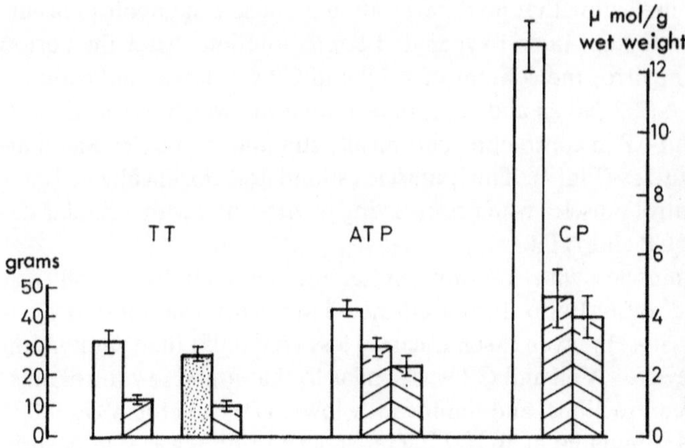

Fig. 7. Twitch tension (in g) and content of ATP and CP (in µmol/g wet weight) in control and chronically stimulated rat EDL muscles at rest and contracting in vitro. □, control muscles at rest; ▨, control muscles contracting; ▩, chronically stimulated muscles at rest; ▧, chronically stimulated muscles contracting

(Gale and Nagle 1971). The decrease in creatinphosphate (from 11.87 ± 0.79 µmol/g wet weight to 4.3 ± 0.74) was also significantly greater ($P < 0.005$) than in chronically stimulated muscles (from 10.8 ± 0.28 to 6.68 ± 0.23 µmol/g wet weight) (Fig. 5).

The initial tension developed by control muscles in vitro after 10 min of equilibration in Krebs solution was similar to that in muscles in vivo (31 ± 3.9 g as opposed to 33 ± 44 g); when the muscles were not contracting, the tension changed very little after another 3–4 min. The decrease in tension during a period of contractions was significantly greater ($P < 0.005$) than in muscles contracting in vivo in both groups – to 36 ± 6.2% in 12 control muscles and to 37.7 ± 5.1% in 7 chronically stimulated muscles (Figs. 6 and 7).

The content of ATP and CP was not different in control resting muscles in vitro from the values found in muscles in vivo (4.25 ± 0.29 µmol/g wet weight for ATP as

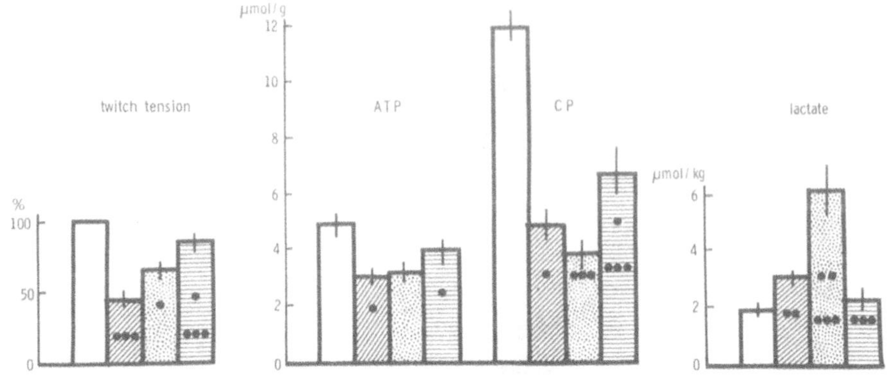

Fig. 8. Twitch tension (TT), content of ATP, creatin phosphate and lactate in rat extensor digitorum longus stimulated for 7 days at 10 Hz ▤ or 40 Hz, 36000 impulses/h, ▩, at the end of 5-min contractions at 4 Hz. ▨, control muscles contracting; □, control muscles at rest. •$P<0.05$, ••$P<0.005$, •••$P<0.001$

opposed to 4.88 ± 0.13 in vivo and 12.9 ± 0.79 µmol/g wet weight for CP as opposed to 11.87 ± 0.79 in vivo) indicating that no deterioration in muscle metabolism occurred when the muscles were kept in an oxygenated Krebs solution. After the period of muscle contractions in vitro, the content of ATP and CP was lower and comparable to that found in vivo (2.7 ± 0.25 and 4.7 ± 0.38 µmol/g wet weight respectively), and the content ATP and CP in contracting chronically stimulated muscles was similar to that in control muscles (Fig. 7). Thus, muscles stimulated chronically at 10 Hz fatigued similarly to control muscles when contracting in vitro, and with a similar decrease in the content of CP and ATP.

Stimulation of rat muscles with intermittent tetanic contractions (3 trains at 40 Hz/min each of 5-s duration) also decreased their fatigability when tested by 5-min twitch contractions at 4 Hz, even if significantly less ($P<0.05$) than stimulation at 10 Hz (Fig. 8). The level of ATP and CP was similar to that found in control muscles at the end of 5 min contractions, and significantly lower ($P<0.05$ for ATP, 0.001 for CP) than in muscles stimulated at 10 Hz. Lactate concentration was significantly higher than in control contracting muscles ($P<0.005$) or muscles that had been stimulated at 10 Hz ($P<0.001$). Although we have no data on the levels of glycogen, it is possible that 40-Hz stimulation depletes glycogen more than 10 Hz, as was shown by Houston et al. (1982) in human muscles stimulated acutely for an hour either intermittently at 50 Hz or continuously at 10 Hz. Galbo et al. (1979) described a correlation between the initial size of glycogen store and lactate production during sustained contractions, and both sets of data would explain the higher increase in lactate concentration in muscles chronically stimulated at 40 Hz.

Conclusions

Chronic electrical stimulation induces capillary growth in different fast muscles in rabbits, rats und cats, whether applied at a frequency occurring naturally in nerves to slow muscles (10 Hz continuously) or with trains of tetanic contractions, provided the total number of impulses is similar and the duration of stimulation is long enough (at least 14 days). The increase in C:F ratio does not seem to be related to the original composition of muscles, as it was greater in rabbit medial gastrocnemius with almost 60% of oxidative fibres than in cat gracilis with 72% of glycolytic fibres. The composition of muscle fibres seems, however, to be important for the changes occurring in the early stages of stimulation. While continuous 10 Hz stimulation induced capillary growth in rabbit and rat EDL before the appearance of any changes in fibre composition, rabbit TA (which is slightly more oxidative) showed an increase in the proportion of oxidative and decreased proportion of glycolytic fibres before the appearance of capillary growth. Stimulation with trains of tetanic contractions increased the proportion of oxidative fibres in rabbit and rat muscles before the appearance of capillary growth. Both types of stimulation improve the resistance to fatigue due to a number of changes occurring with prolonged stimulation (Hudlická et al. 1982b; Pette and Vrbová 1985). The reasons for this improvement might be different at the early stages of stimulation. Increased capillary supply seems to be of primary importance for improved muscle performance due to improved rephosphorylation of ATP and CP in muscles stimulated at 10 Hz, while increased activity of oxidative enzymes and changes in glycogen metabolism probably play a role in those stimulated at 40 Hz.

References

Aitman TJ, Hudlická O, Tyler KR (1979) Long-term effects of tetanic stimulation on blood flow, metabolism and performance of fast skeletal muscles. J Physiol 295:36–37P

Ariano MA, Armstrong RB, Edgerton VR (1973) Hind-limb muscle fibre populations of five mammals. J Histochem Cytochem 21:51–55

Bass A, Brdiczka D, Eyer P, Hofer S, Pette D (1969) Metabolic differentiation of distinct muscle types at the level of enzymatic organization. Eur J Biochemi 10:198–206

Brånemark PI (1965) Capillary form and function. Bibl Anat 7:9–28

Brooke MH, Kaiser KK (1969) Some comments on the histochemical characterization of muscle adenosine triphosphatase. J Histochem Cytochem 17:431–432

Brown MD, Cotter MA, Hudlická O, Vrbová G (1976) The effects of different patterns of muscle activity on capillary density, mechanical properties and structure of slow and fast rabbit muscles. Pflugers Arch 361:241–250

Cotter M, Hudlická O, Vrbová G (1973) Growth of capillaries during long-term activity in skeletal muscle. Bibl Anat 11:395–398

Dawson J, Hudlická O, Tyler KR (1983) Measurement of flow velocities in capillaries supplying fast and slow muscle fibres at rest and during contractions in the rat. J Physiol 338:7P

Galbo H, Holst JJ, Christensen NJ (1979) The effect of different diets and of insulin on the hormonal response to prolonged exercise. Acta Physiol Scand 107:19–32

Gale JB, Nagle FY (1971) Changes in ATP and creatinphosphate storage in skeletal muscles of rats trained at 900 and 7600 feet. Nature 232:342

Gray SD, Renkin EM (1978) Microvascular supply in relation to fiber metabolic type in mixed skeletal muscles of rabbit. Microvasc Res 16:406–425

Hoppeler H, Mathieu O, Weibel ER, Krauer R, Lindstedt SL, Taylor CR (1981) Design of the mammalian respiratory system. VIII Capillaries in skeletal muscle. Respir Physiol 44:129–150

Hoppeler H, Hudlická O, Uhlmann E (1983) The relationship between capillary density, volume density of mitochondria and maximal blood flow in various cat muscles. J Physiol 342:32P

Houston ME, Farrance BW, Wight RI (1982) Metabolic effects of two frequencies of short-term surface electrical stimulation on human muscle. Can J Physiol Pharmacol 60:727–731

Hudlická O (1982) Growth of capillaries in skeletal and cardiac muscle. Circ Res 50:451–461
Hudlická O (1985) Development and adaptability of microvasculature in skeletal muscle. J Exp Biol 115:319–331
Hudlická O, el Khelly F (1985) Metabolic factors involved in regulation of muscle blood flow. J Cardiovasc Pharmacol [Suppl] 3:559–572
Hudlická O, Schroeder W (1978) Factors involved in capillary growth in a normal adult skeletal muscle (abstract). Fed Proc 37:314
Hudlická O, Tyler KR (1984) The effect of long-term high-frequency stimulation on capillary density and fibre types in rabbit fast muscles. J Physiol 353:435–445
Hudlická O, Brown M, Cotter M, Smith M, Vrbová G (1977) The effect of long-term stimulation of fast muscles on their blood flow, metabolism and ability to withstand fatigue. Pflugers Arch 369:141–149
Hudlická O, Dodd L, Renkin EM, Gray SD (1982a) Early changes in fiber profiles and capillary density in long-term stimulated muscles. Am J Physiol 243:H528–535
Hudlická O, Tyler KR, Srihari T, Heilig A, Pette D (1982b) The effect of different patterns of long-term stimulation on contractile properties and myosing light chains in rabbit fast muscles. Pflugers Arch 393:164–170
Hudlická O, Aitman T, Heilig A, Leberer E, Tyler KR, Pette D (1984) Effects of different patterns of long-term stimulation on blood flow, fuel uptake and enzyme activities in rabbit fast skeletal muscles. Pflugers Arch 402:306–311
Kanabus EW, Hudlická O, Tyler KR (1980) Skeletal muscle PO_2 after chronic tetanic stimulation. Microvasc Res 20:113–114
Mathieu O, Cruz-Orive L-M, Hoppeler H, Weibel ER (1983) Estimating length density and quantifying anisotrophy in skeletal muscle capillaries. J Microsc 131:131–146
Myrhage R, Hudlická O (1976) The microvascular bed and capillary surface area in rat extensor hallucis proprius muscle (EHP). Microvasc Res 11:315–323
Myrhage R, Hudlická O (1978) Capillary growth in chronically stimulated adult skeletal muscle as studied by intravital microscopy and histological methods in rabbits and rats. Microvasc Res 16:73–90
Pearse AGE (1968) Histochemistry-theoretical and applied, 3rd ed., vol 1. Churchill, London
Pette D, Tyler KR (1983) Response of succinate dehydrogenase activity in fibres of rabbit tibialis anterior muscle to chronic nerve stimulation. J Physiol 338:1–9
Pette D, Vrbová G (1985) Neural control of phenotype expression in mammalian muscle fiber. Muscle Nerve 8:676–689
Pette D, Smith ME, Staudte HW, Vrbová G (1973) Effect of long-term electrical stimulation on some contractile metabolic characteristics of fast rabbit muscles. Pflugers Arch 338:257–272
Pette D, Ramirez BU, Muller W, Simon R, Exner GU, Hildebrand R (1975) Influence of intermittent stimulation on contractile, histochemical and metabolic properties of fibre populations in fast and slow rabbit muscles. Pflugers Arch 361:1–7
Pette D, Muller W, Leisner E, Vrbová G (1976) Time dependent effects on contractile properties, fiber population, myosin light chains and enzymes of energy metabolism in intermittently and continuously stimulated fast-twitch muscles of the rabbit. Pflugers Arch 364:103–112
Ranvier L (1874) Note sur les vaisseaux sanguins et la circulation dans les muscles rouges. CR Soc Biol (Paris) 26:28–31
Romanul FCA (1965) Capillary supply and metabolism of muscle fibers. Arch Neurol 12:497–509
Salmons S, Vrbová G (1969) The influence of activity on some contractile characteristics of mammalian fast and slow muscles. J Physiol 201:535–549
Thoma R (1911) Über die Histomechanik des Gefäßsystems und die Pathogenese der Angiosklerose. Virchows Archiv [A] 204:1–74
Waxman AM (1981) Blood vessel growth as a problem in morphogenesis: a physical theory. Microvasc Res 22:32–41

The Acetylcholine Receptor and Neural Control of Its Distribution

F. Vyskočil[1]

Acetylcholine Receptor

The nicotinic acetylcholine (ACh) receptor (AChR) is to date the best characterized protein involved in synaptic communication [see Cold Spring Harbor Symposia (1983) and the excellent reviews by Barrantes et al. (1983) and Popot and Changeux (1984)]. In a pure form, large amounts of AChR can be isolated (100 mg AChR protein per kg tissue) from the sea ray *Torpedo* or from eel *Electrophorus* electroplaques either in its native membrane-bound state or by affinity chromatography after solubilization. At the neuromuscular junction, receptors of the muscle postsynaptic membrane are packed in paracrystalline array "rosettes" with a density which exceeds their density elsewhere on the muscle cell by several orders of magnitude (Fambrough 1979). The AChR-rich regions (clusters) of the muscle fibre membrane are not continuous but are divided by AChR-poor regions. In many species, the post-synaptic membrane is enfolded and the ACh-rich regions form a crest of the folds and the AChR-free regions are in their depth (Fertuck and Salpeter 1976).

It is now well established that monomeric AChR with a molecular weight of about 300000 (Lo et al. 1981) has a complex subunit structure and is composed of four different proteins. They have about 500 amino acids and apparent molecular weights of 39000, 48000, 58000 and 64000 in *Torpedo californica* and are commonly referred to as α, β, γ and δ respectively (see e.g. Conti-Tronconti and Raftery 1982) in the stoichiometry α_2, β, γ, and δ (Reynolds and Karlin 1978; Lindstrom et al. 1979a; Raftery et al. 1980). Each chain of the native receptor is glycosylated. The subunits are very similar in general structure and have homologous stretches which contain nearly the same amino acids. Each protomer spans the membrane and five of them are arranged in a rosette to form a central pore through which ions flow (see Stevens 1985). The receptor isolated from the *Torpedo* electric organ exists in dimeric and monomeric form. The dimeric state of the receptor predominates in the intact membrane and depends upon sulphydryl interactions between the δ chains (Karlin et al. 1979) and on the 43000 peptide located on the inner side of the membrane (Barrantes 1982). Karlin et al. (1979) suggested that self-association of receptor units might play a role in the formation of receptor clusters within the membrane.

Venoms of the krait *Bungarus multicintus* and cobras of the *Naja* species contain an α-toxin which acts as a specific and (almost) irreversible competitor of ACh for the receptor. Quantitative binding of α-bungarotoxin (α-BnTX) to the intact membrane allowed the estimation of 18000 toxin binding sites per μm^2 of the membrane surface at the peaks of the endplate folds (Albuquerque et al. 1974; Fertuck and

1 Institute of Physiology, Czechoslovak Academy of Sciences, Prague, Czechoslovakia

Electrical Stimulation and Neuromuscular Disorders
Ed. by W. A. Nix and G. Vrbová

Salpeter 1976; Land et al. 1980). Because there is evidence that α-bungarotoxin forms a bond specifically to the α-chain (Karlin et al. 1975) of which there are two per receptor, the maximum density of the AChR is about $9000/\mu m^2$. The density of the AChR – together with single channel conductance – determines the degree of sensitivity to ACh (Albuquerque et al. 1974) and to some extent the rate of rise of the ACh responses (Land et al. 1980; Dwyer et al. 1981). Binding of α-toxin has also enabled a detailed evaluation of the life span of the AChR (Devreotes and Fambrough 1975; Fambrough 1983; Linden and Fambrough 1979). A number of topical reviews have placed emphasis on AChR function (Changeux 1981; Conti-Troconti and Raftery 1982; Barrantes 1983; Anholt et al. 1984; Lambert et al. 1983; Maelicke and Prinz 1983; Peper et al. 1982; Spivak and Albuquerque 1982; Taylor and Sine 1981) structure (Cartaud et al. 1980; Hamilton 1982; Wennogle 1985; Karlin 1983; Stroud 1983; Popot and Changeux 1984) and functional reconstitution in artificial lipid bilayers (Anholt et al. 1983; McNamee and Ochoa 1982; Popot 1983) and on clonical studies of patients with the autoimmune disease myasthenia gravis (Vincent 1980; Grob 1981; Drachman 1981; Lindstrøm 1983).

AChR is thus defined as a rather nonspecific ion channel for Na^+, K^+, and Ca^{2+}, operated by ACh. Many studies (see the listed reviews) indicate that the α-subunits carry binding sites for ACh, that the β- and δ-subunits probably take part in the supramolecular organisation of the postsynaptic membrane, that at least the γ- and δ-subunits carry phosphorylation sites and that all subunits contribute to the formation of the transmembrane channel. The five subunits are probably arranged around the central pit in the order $\alpha\gamma\alpha\beta\delta$. Opening and closing of the channel may involve concerted conformational transitions of a part, if not all, of the receptor channel complex. As has been stressed by Popot and Changeux (1984), the spatial relationship between the various sites and the identity of the intersubunit interfaces involved in propagating conformational transitions depend on the exact arrangement of the subunits within the oligomer. In their review (Popot and Changeux 1984), the overall structural model of fish AChR molecule is presented (p. 1222) which only differs slightly from the three dimensional model of Stroud and co-workers (see Stroud 1983).

Some 10–15 years ago, physiologists were still unsure whether the recognition site of the receptor and the pore through which the ions move are really part of the same molecule (e.g. Magazanik and Vyskočil 1973, 1976). Now it is clear that they are, and this information was obtained by a new technique, the patch clamp, for recording the movement of ions through a single channel. This was achieved on the basis of Erwin Neher's observation in 1979 that a very tight seal develops when suction is applied to a heat-polished 2–3 μm glass pipette placed against a cell membrane. The perfect electrical and mechanical isolation of a small piece of membrane under the pipette with only one or a few channels operated by voltage or by transmitters permits the use of a larger variety of procedures and experimental conditions than was previously possible (Hamill et al. 1981; Sakmann and Neher 1983).

Magleby and Stevens (1972) suggested a model where ACh molecules which bind to the receptor initiate fast channel opening of a few milliseconds on the average; closing of the channel is slower. After the channel closes, ACh unbinds rapidly and diffuses away. According to this model, AChR exists only in two states – closed or open. It was also established that two ACh molecules must normally form a bond for the channel to open (Adams 1975; Dionne et al. 1978). Although the Magleby-Stevens model is correct in principle, patch clamp studies on single AChR-channels revealed that there are two open states, longer and shorter. It is possible that the shorter (less than 1 ms) represents channels opening with a single ACh molecule bound while the longer open time (about 10 ms) represents a more stable opening with two ACh molecules (Colquhoun and Sakmann 1981). Another observation, obtained with the patch clamp technique, was that these opening are actually interrupted by very brief 50-μs closings (flickering or the *Nachschlag*) before the final closing (Colquhoun and Sakmann 1981; Dionne and Leibowitz 1982). Furthermore, AChR have been observed to enter a state where only about a third of the normal current flows (Hamill and Sakmann 1981a; Trautmann 1982). This "substate" in principle negates the basic presumption of channel kinetics, namely that biological channels have a single fixed conductance for all open states. It is clear now – and this applies also for several other membrane ionic channels – that they can have several different conductances. The last important behaviour of the AChR channel is that the current record is more noisy when the channel is open than when it is closed. This may be explained by quivering of the channel protein caused by motion of neighbouring water or lipid molecules when the channel pore region changes in dimension.

Innervation and AChR Properties

In 1967, Beránek and Vyskočil found that 1–2 weeks after denervation, the extrajunctional response (Ginetzinski and Shamarina 1942) of rat diaphragm muscle fibres to iontophoretically applied ACh was less sensitive to the blockade with curare than that of the innervated end-plate. This pharmacological difference was confirmed and other workers showed that the cholinergic ligands curare, carbamylcholine and decamethonium were less effective in protecting denervation-induced extrasynaptic AChR from binding of α-BuTX (Berg et al. 1972; Chiu et al. 1973; Porter et al. 1973; Lapa et al. 1974; Sarvey et al. 1978). Almon and Appel (1975) showed that the antibody from myasthenia gravis patients did not protect junctional rat receptors from binding the α-toxin, whereas it did protect the denervation-induced AChR as well as those of normal human muscle. It is now clear that the neuromuscular form of AChR shows two distinct subsets, junctional and extrajunctional. These two types of channel differ in density (Michler and Sakmann 1980), kinetics of α-toxin binding (Lo et al. 1981), receptor metabolism (Berg and Hall 1975a, b; Michler and Sakmann 1980) immunologic reactivity (Almon and Appel 1976), translational diffusion coefficient (Axelrod et al. 1976), gating kinetics (Katz and Miledi 1972; Sakmann and Brenner 1978; Fischbach and Schuetze 1980) and noise-inferred conductance (Neher and Sakmann 1976a). The differences between AChR located junctionally and newly synthesized (Devreotes and Fambrough 1975) extrajunctional receptors can be attributed not only to different affinities for cholinergic ligands but also to the metabolic stability which decreases after denervation (Loring and Salpeter 1980; Stanley and Drachman 1981). The differences in intrinsic receptor properties were indicated by Brockes and Hall (1975). They reported that the isoelectric point of denervation-induced extrajunctional AChR was 0.15 pH units higher than that of normal junctional receptors. This may, for example, reflect the degree of phosphorylation and dephosphorylation of receptor subunits (Teichberg and Changeux 1976) or shift in subunit composition (see below). At 7–14 days after denervation, the former end-plate region of the rat diaphragm possessed a heterogenous population of AChR with regard to the isoelectric point and mean opening time, the latter being at least twice as long for denervated muscle AChR (Dreyer et al. 1976; Neher and Sakmann 1976a). The heterogeneity is apparently due to the persistence of pre-denervation receptors (Levitt et al. 1980) at the post-junctional membrane. Furthermore, the conductance of extrajunctional AChR is lower than the junctional one by 30%–50% (17 and 8 pS, Dreyer et al. 1976; or 23 and 15 pS, Neher and Sakmann 1976a). Thus, the extrajunctional AChR allows less ions to pass but remains open longer than the junctional system (Katz and Miledi 1972; Dreyer et al. 1976). This may be due to a denervation-induced change in the charge distribution within the channel, alterations in membrane composition or the total transmembrane electric field (McArdle 1983). The extrajunctional receptors (perijunctional as well as those induced by denervation) are considered to be identical, or at least very similar, to embryonal receptors and those at early postnatal periods. Sakmann and Brenner (1978) found that in the soleus neuromuscular junction of the rat, the mean channel opening time was 3.9 ms on day 8 and 1.0 ms on day 18 after birth.

End-plate current analysis (noise spectra and the decay of miniature end-plate currents) showed that there are two populations of receptors with a slow and a fast decaying component. The contribution (probably the number) of the slow state AChR decreases until, at 18 days, the fast type completely prevails (see also Schuetze and Fischbach 1978; Fischbach and Schuetze 1980). As a possible explanation of the differences in channel properties occurring during maturation of the receptor system, one can consider, for example, the posttranslational modification or synthesis of a new protein. The latter possibility is favoured by recent findings of Noda, Numa and co-workers (Takai et al. 1985). These authors (after successfully elucidating the primary structure of all four subunits of the *Torpedo,* calf muscle and α- and γ-subunits of human muscle AChR) cloned DNA complementary to foetal calf muscle mRNA encoding a novel polypeptide, the ε-subunit, whose deduced amino-acid sequence has features characteristic of other subunits and a high sequence homology to the γ-subunit. To examine whether the ε-subunit can function as an AChR subunit, they synthetized the mRNA specific for this protein in vitro, using the cDNA template and injected the mRNA together with α-, β- and δ-subunit specific mRNA into oocytes of the frog *Xenopus.* The treated oocytes developed AChR of the nicotinic type. The authors speculate that the ε-subunit (and probably the γ-subunit as well) may be a decisive component of the extrajunctional type of AChR. On the other hand, the ε-subunit contains more acidic residues and less basic residues than the γ-subunit. But, if it were this subunit which is characteristic of extrajunctional AChR, one should, according to Nathanson and Hall (1979), expect it to be more alkaline and less acidic. This recent example demonstrates that neurologists will soon be informed about subtle molecular differences in AChR and about their regulation at the genetic level in experimental animals as well as in man.

AChRs are not only altered during maturation or denervation, but their functional properties (and probably also their number) may change in muscles of adult animals. Desensitization (progressive loss of AChR functional sensitivity to ACh during longlasting exposure to the agonist, Thesleff 1955; Katz and Thesleff 1957; Magazanik and Vyskočil 1970, 1973, 1975) is an all-or-none channel process due to a progressive conversion of a number or of all AChRs to the closed, non-operable state with a higher affinity for the agonist (Sakmann et al. 1980; Gration et al. 1981). The onset and recovery of this process does not substantially change after denervation (Vyskočil 1975; Colquhoun and Rang 1976) (although Hall et al. 1977 expressed an opposite view). The longlasting presence of ACh around the AChR leads to the desensitization process which is biphasic with a fast and a slow component (Feltz and Trautmann 1982). There are a number of factors which control desensitization; for example, its onset is promoted by higher polarization of the muscle cell (Magazanik and Vyskočil 1970; Scubon-Mulieri and Parsons 1978), higher temperature (Magazanik and Vyskočil 1975) and many different chemicals, including detergents, anaesthetics, psychotrophic drugs such as chlorpromazine (Magazanik et al. 1982) or diazepam (Vyskočil 1978). According to Akasu and Karczmar (1980) NaF protects the frog AChR from desensitization.

An important question is whether desensitization has any influence upon synaptic transmission. Thesleff (1959) first suggested this possibility, but more recently, Magleby and Pallotta (1981) demonstrated that the ACh released during nerve stimulation of several minutes' duration reduce the single quantal responses in the frog endplate. Desensitization may also contribute to neuromuscular transmission failure in myasthenia gravis (Pagala et al. 1981, 1982). The steady activation of the end-plate membrane might occur (after anticholineterase poisoning in particular) due to nonquantal, molecular leakage of ACh (Katz and Miledi 1977b; Vyskočil and Illés 1977, 1978; Vyskočil et al. 1983; Edwards et al. 1985) which accounts for more than 95% of the overall amount of ACh released at rest (Fletcher and Forrester 1975; Gorio et al. 1978; Vizi and Vyskočil 1979; Polak et al. 1981). This process may lead to the lowering of the number of receptor sites. The agonist-induced loss of AChR was observed in vitro (Klein et al. 1976; Gardner and Fambrough 1979; Messing 1982) as well as in vivo (Taylor et al. 1982).

The role of muscle activity in the regulation of AChR distribution has been experimentally demonstrated. Despite the fact that Johns and Thesleff (1961) found that spinalization does not result in hypersensitivity to ACh in the cat, and that the partially denervated "two junctional" frog muscle fibres could become hypersensitive even if they are still physiologically active, Lømo and Rosenthal (1972) showed clearly that AChR extrajunctional distribution and two other main membrane properties (resting membrane potential which drops significantly after denervation and fibre cable properties such as specific membrane resistance which is elevated in denervated muscles) are altered with activity. Among other observations, they showed that after chronic stimulation of denervated rat muscles, the extrajunctional ACh sensitivity was greatly reduced or even abolished. In 1975, Lømo and Westgaard, like Purves and Sakmann (1974), demonstrated that the reduction of postdenervation AChR depends strongly on the pattern of stimulation. Brief trains of 100-Hz pulses were more effective than stimuli applied at a low frequency. Nevertheless, only activity itself cannot be fully responsible for alterations in AChR distribution as well as for changes in other membrane parameters. Lavoie et al. (1976, 1977) implanted tetrodotoxin containing plastic cuffs around the nerve; this elimination of activity (without interference in axoplasmic flow) elevated α-toxin binding to the muscle but its magnitude was less than that seen after denervation. Similarly, complete inactivation of embryonic and cultured muscles does not abolish AChR clustering (Braithwaite and Harris 1979; Steinbach 1974). On the contrary, stimulation of denervated muscles in vitro lowers but does not completely prevent the synthesis of the receptor (Hogan et al. 1976; Hall and Reiness 1977). However, Desphande et al. (1976) pointed out that the denervated muscle is a pathologically altered organ and hence cannot serve as a model for studying neural influences on normal muscles. Chronic stimulation of denervated muscles decreases that AChR extrajunctional receptor formation but, at the same time, also depresses the mechanical responses of muscles (Purves and Sakmann 1974; Linden and Fambrough 1979). This may imply a shift in the proteins which the stimulated muscle is synthesizing (McArdle 1983). Thesleff and Sellin (1980) published an apt diagram showing the denervated muscle as a factory for AChR production. Stimulation may then force the "factory" to produce a different protein to meet the new demands. This might, according to McArdle (1983), occur at the expense of the AChR, since the materials and energy available to the denervated muscle may be limited.

The regulation of AChR synthesis and distribution cannot be considered separately from the overall consideration of neurotrophic relations (Gutmann 1976) and normal functional activity, which is, as a rule, the plastic complex resulting from the particular functional role of the given muscle in the organism.

In his exhaustive review, McArdle (1983) attempted to list the most common events and biochemical pathways involved in normal functional activity of skeletal muscle fibres. These are – with slight modification – as follows: 1) binding of ACh to the receptor, 2) AChR channel opening, 3) Na^+, K^+ (and CA^{2+}) fluxes underlying local end-plate potential, 4) voltage sensitive channel opening for Na^+ and then for K^+-action potential, 5) subsequent restoration of the Na^+-K^+ gradient via the pump, 6) release of Ca^{2+} from the sarcoplasmic reticulum, 7) activation of actin-myosin ATPase, 8) shortening of the muscle fibre, 9) uptake of Ca^{2+} into the sarcoplasmic reticulum, 10) uptake of Ca^{2+} into mitochondria and coupled electron transport.

It is clear that the ACh-AChR interaction and pumping of ions are important. But other functional steps may also fulfil regulatory functions. Gruener et al. (1974) pointed out that subthreshold electrical stimulation – without evoking action potentials and muscle shortening – is capable of lowering postdenervation AChR synthesis, and Powell and Friedman (1977) showed that skeletal muscles in muscular dysgenesis mutant mice may exhibit spontaneous action potentials "in vitro" without contraction, but also without postdenervation AChR induction. Thus, propagated and non-propagated electrical activity alone is sufficient to control the AChR number, and mechanical shortening is apparently not necessary. Under normal conditions, localized currents develop in muscle. The end-plate zone of fibres of twitch skeletal muscles is hyperpolarized by 1–3 mV as compared with extrajunctional regions (Vyskočil 1974; Vyskočil and Illés 1978). This might be the result of activation of Na^+-K^+ ATPase by ACh (or choline?) at this zone (Dlouhá et al. 1979). Betz et al. (1980) found that localized end-plate currents are inhibited by ouabain. It is therefore probable that the molecular release of ACh may modulate muscle fibre resting electrogenesis and by exerting this control to modify, to a certain extent, AChR distribution (Sun and Poo 1985).

Despite the great progress in our knowledge of the biochemistry and gene expression of AChR, many regulatory influences such as non-impulse nerve-mediated factors (Vyskočil and Gutmann 1976; Vyskočil et al. 1981), other neurotrophic molecules (Thoenen et al. 1983), basal lamina (Nitkin et al. 1983) and other diverse interactions occur at neuromuscular junction, which is a morphologically and functionally plastic zone. We ought therefore still to agree with Ernest Gutmann who wrote ten years ago that "regulation of ACh receptors is a complex process and differentiation of the components is not yet achieved" (Gutmann 1976).

Acknowledgement. The author is grateful to Dr. Pavel Hník and Mrs. Jarmila Hýžová for their help during the preparation of the manuscript.

References

Adams PR (1975) An analysis of the dose-response curve at voltage-clamped frog endplates. Pflugers Arch 360:145–153

Akasu T, Karczmar AG (1980) Effects of anticholinesterases and of sodium fluoride on neuromyal desensitization. Neuropharmacol 19:393–403

Albuquerque EX, Barnard EA, Porter CW, Warnick JE (1974) The density of acetylcholine receptors and their sensitivity in the postsynaptic membrane of muscle end-plates. Proc Natl Acad Sci USA 71:2818–2822

Almon RR, Appel SH (1975) Interaction of myasthenic serum globulin with the acetylcholine receptor. Biochim Biophys Acta 393:66–77

Almon RR, Appel SH (1976) Cholinergic sites in skeletal muscle. I. Denervation effects. Biochemistry 15:3662–3667

Anholt R, Montal M, Lindstrøm J (1983) Incorporation of acetylcholine receptors in model membranes: an approach aimed at studies of the molecular basis of neurotransmission. In: Hearn M (ed) Peptide and protein reviews, vol 1. Dekker, New York, pp 95–137

Anholt R, Lindstrøm J, Montal M (1984) The molecular basis of neurotransmission: structure and function of the nicotinic acetylcholine receptor. In: Martonosi A (ed) The enzymes of biological membranes, vol 3. Plenum, New York, pp 335–401

Axelrod D, Ravdin P, Koppel DE, Schlessinger J, Webb WW, Elson EL, Podleski TR (1976) Lateral motion of fluorescently labeled acetylcholine receptors in membranes of developing muscle fibers. Proc Natl Acad Sci USA 73:4594–4598

Barrantes FJ (1982) Oligomeric forms of the membrane-bound acetylcholine receptor disclosed upon extraction of the M, 43000 non-receptor peptide. J Cell Biol 92:60–68

Barrantes FJ (1983) Recent developments in the structure and function of the acetylcholine receptor. Int Rev Neurobiol 24:259–341

Barrantes FJ, Mieskes G, Wallimann T (1983) Creatine-kinase activity in the *Torpedo* electrocyte and in the non-receptor, peripheral γ-proteins from acetylcholine receptor-rich membranes. Proc Natl Acad Sci USA 80:5440–5444

Beránek R, Vyskočil F (1967) The action of tubocurarine and atropine on the normal and denervated rat diaphragm. J Physiol (Lond) 188:53–66

Berg DK, Hall ZW (1975a) Increased extrajunctional acetylcholine sensitivity produced by chronic post-synaptic neuromuscular blockade. J Physiol (Lond) 244:659–676

Berg DK, Hall ZW (1975b) Loss of alpha-bungarotoxin from junctional and extrajunctional acetylcholine receptors in rat diaphragm muscle in vivo and in organ culture. J Physiol (Lond) 252:771–789

Berg DK, Kelly RB, Sargent PB, Williamson P, Hall Z (1972) Binding of alpha-bungarotoxin to acetylcholine receptors in mammalian muscle. Proc Natl Acad Sci USA 69:147–151

Betz WJ, Caldwell JH, Ribchester RR, Robinson KR, Stump RF (1980) Endogenous electric field around muscle fibres is dependent on the Na^+-K^+ pump. Nature 287:235–237

Braithwaite AW, Harris AJ (1979) Neural influence on acetylcholine receptor clusters in embryonic development of skeletal muscles. Nature 279:549–551

Brockes JP, Hall ZW (1975) Acetylcholine receptors in normal and denervated rat diaphragm muscle. II. Comparison of junctional and extrajunctional receptors. Biochemistry 14:2100–2106

Cartaud J, Popot JL, Changeux JP (1980) Light and heavy forms of the acetylcholine receptor from *Torpedo marmorata* electric organ: morphological identification using reconstituted vesicles. FEBS Lett 121:327–332

Changeux JP (1981) The acetylcholine receptor: an "allosteric" membrane protein. Harvey Lectures, vol 75. Academic, New York, pp 85–254

Chiu TH, Dolly JO, Barnard EA (1973) Solubilization from skeletal muscle of two components that specifically bind alphabungarotoxin. Biochem Biophys Res Commun 51:205–213

Cold Spring Harbor Symposia on Quantitative Biology (1983) Vol 48: Molecular neurobiology. Cold Spring Harbor Laboratory, New York

Colquhoun D, Rang HP (1976) Effects of inhibitors on the binding of ionated alpha-bungarotoxin to acetylcholine receptors in rat muscle. Mol Pharmacol 12:519–535

Colquhoun D, Sakmann B (1981) Fluctuations in the microsecond time range of the current through single acetylcholine receptor ion channels. Nature 294:464–466

Conti-Troconti BM, Raftery MA (1982) The nicotinic cholinergic receptor: correlation of molecular structure with functional properties. Annu Rev Biochem 51:491–530

Desphande SS, Albuquerque EX, Guth L (1976) Neurotrophic regulation of prejunctional and postjunctional membrane at the mammalian motor end-plate. Exp Neurol 53:151–165

Devreotes PN, Fambrough DM (1975) Acetylcholine receptor turnover in membrane of developing muscle fibers. J Cell Biol 65:335–358

Dionne VE, Leibowitz MD (1982) Acetylcholine receptor kinetics: A description from single-channel currents at snake neuromuscular junctions. Biophys J 39:253–261

Dionne VE, Steinbach JH, Stevens CF (1978) An analysis of the dose-response relationship at voltage-clamped frog neuromuscular junction. J Physiol 281:421–444

Dlouhá H, Teisinger J, Vyskočil F (1979) Activation of Na^+/K^+-ATPase of mouse skeletal muscle by acetylcholine and its inhibition by alpha-bungarotoxin, curare and atropine. Pflugers Arch 380:101–104

Drachman D (1981) The biology of myasthenia gravis. Ann Rev Neurosci 4:195–225

Dreyer F, Müller Peper K, Sterz R (1976) The M. Omohyoideus of the mouse as a convenient mammalian muscle preparation. A study of junctional and extrajunctional acetylcholine receptors by noise analysis and cooperativy. Pflugers Arch 367:115–122

Dwyer D, Kearney J, Bradley R, Kemp G, Oh S (1981) Interaction of human antibody and murine monoclonal antibody with muscle acetylcholine receptor. Ann NY Acad Sci 377:143–157

Edwards C, Doležal V, Tuček S, Zemková H, Vyskočil F (1985) Is an acetylcholine transport system responsible for nonquantal release of acetylcholine at the rodent myoneural junction? Proc Natl Acad Sci USA 82:3514–3518

Fambrough DM (1979) Control of acetylcholine receptors in skeletal muscle. Physiol Rev 59:165–227

Fambrough DM (1983) Biosynthesis and intracellular transport of acetylcholine receptors. In: Fleischer S, Fleischer B (eds) Methods in enzymology, vol 96: biomembranes-membrane biogenesis: assembly and targeting (general methods, eukaryotes). Academic, New York, pp 331–352

Feltz A, Trautmann A (1982) Desensitization of the frog neuromuscular junction: a biphasic process. J Physiol (Lond) 322:257–272

Fertuck HC, Salpeter MM (1976) Quantitation of junctional and extrajunctional acetylcholine receptors by electron microscope autoradiography after ^{125}I-alpha-bungarotoxin binding at mouse neuromuscular junctions. J Cell Biol 69:144–158

Fischbach GD, Schuetze SM (1980) A post-natal decrease in acetylcholine channel open time of rat end-plates. J Physiol (Lond) 303:125–137

Fletcher P, Forrester T (1975) The effect of curare on the release of acetylcholine from mammalian motor nerve terminals and an estimate of quantal content. J Physiol (Lond) 251:131–144

Gardner JM, Fambrough DM (1979) Acetylcholine receptor degradation measured by density labeling: effects of cholinergic ligands and evidence against recycling. Cell 16:661–674
Ginetzinski AG, Shamarina NM (1942) The tonomotor phenomenon in denervated muscles. Usp Sovrem Biol 15:283–294 (in Russian)
Gorio A, Hurlbut WP, Ceccarelli B (1978) Acetylcholine compartments in mouse diaphragm: a comparison of the effects of black widow spider venom, electrical stimulation and high concentrations of potassium. J Cell Biol 78:716–733
Gration KAF, Lambert JJ, Usherwood PNR (1981) A comparison of glutamate single-channel activity at desensitizing and nondesensitizing sites. J Physiol (Lond) 310:49P
Grob D (ed) (1981) Myasthenia gravis: pathology and management. Ann NY Acad Sci 377:1–902
Gruener R, Baumbach N, Doffee D (1974) Reduction of denervation supersensitivity of muscle by submechanical threshold stimulation. Nature 248:68–69
Gutmann E (1976) Neurotrophic relations. Annu Rev Physiol 38:177–216
Hall MT, Maleque MA, Wadsworth RM (1977) The role of extracellular calcium in the contractions produced by acetylcholine in chronically denervated muscle. Br J Pharmacol 61:627–638
Hall ZW, Reiness CG (1977) Electrical stimulation of denervated muscles reduces incorporation of methionine into the ACh receptor. Nature 268:655–657
Hamill OP, Sakmann B (1981a) Multiple conductance states of single acetylcholine receptor channels in embryonic muscle cells. Nature 294:462–464
Hamill OP, Sakmann B (1981b) A cell-free method for recording single-channel currents from biological membranes. J Physiol 312:41P–42P
Hamill OP, Marty A, Neher E, Sakmann B, Sigworth FJ (1981) Improved patch-clamp techniques for high-resolution current recording from cells and cell-free membrane patches. Pflugers Arch 391:85–100
Hamilton SL (1982) The structure of the nicotinic acetylcholine recptor. Prog Clin Biol Res 79:73–85
Hogan PG, Marshall JM, Hall ZW (1976) Muscle activity decreases rate of degradation of alpha-bungarotoxin bound to extrajunctional acetylcholine receptors. Nature 261:328–330
Johns TR, Thesleff S (1961) Effects of motor inactivation on the chemical sensitivity of skeletal muscle. Acta Physiol Scand 51:136–141
Karlin A (1983) The anatomy of a receptor. Neurosci Comment 1:111–123
Karlin A, Weill CL, McNamee MG, Valderamma R (1975) Facets of the structures of acetylcholine receptors from *Electrophorus* and *Torpedo*. Cold Spring Harbor Symp Quant Biol 40:203–210
Karlin A, Damle V, Hamilton S, McLaughlin M, Valderamma R, Wise D (1979) Acetylcholine receptors in and out of membranes. In: Ceccarelli B (ed) Advances in cytopharmacology, vol 3. Raven, New York, pp 183–188
Katz B, Miledi R (1972) The statistical nature of the acetylcholine potential and its molecular components. J Physiol (Lond) 224:665–699
Katz B, Miledi R (1977a) The reversal potential at the desensitized end-plate. Proc R Soc Lond [Biol] 199:329–334
Katz B, Miledi R (1977b) Transmitter leakage from motor nerve endings. Proc R Soc Lond [Biol] 196:59–72
Katz B, Thesleff S (1957) A study of the "desensitization" produced by acetylcholine at the motor end-plate. J Physiol (Lond) 138:63–80
Klein W, Nathanson NM, Nirenberg M (1976) Long-term receptor mediated regulation of acetylcholine receptors and adenylate cyclase in hybrid cells. Fed Am Soc Exp Biol 35:1576 (abstract)
Lambert JJ, Durant NN, Henderson EG (1983) Drug-induced modification of ionic conductance at the neuromuscular junction. Annu Rev Pharmacol Toxicol 23:505–539
Land BR, Salpeter EE, Salpeter MM (1980) Acetylcholine receptor site density affects the rising phase of miniature endplate currents. Proc Natl Acad Sci USA 77:3736–3740
Lapa AJ, Albuquerque EX, Daly J (1974) An electrophysiological study of the effects of d-tubocurarine, atrophine and alpha-bungarotoxin on the cholinergic receptor in innervated and chronically denervated mammalian skeletal muscles. Exp Neurol 43:375–398
Lavoie PA, Collier B, Tenenhouse A (1976) Comparison of alpha-bungarotoxin binding to skeletal muscles after inactivity of denervation. Nature 260:349–350
Lavoie PA, Collier B, Tenenhouse A (1977) Role of skeletal muscle activity in the control of muscle acetylcholine sensitivity. Exp Neurol 54:148–171

Levitt TA, Loring RH, Salpeter MM (1980) Neuronal control of acetylcholine receptor turnover rate a vertebrate neuromuscular junction. Science 210:550–551

Linden DC, Fambrough DM (1979) Biosynthesis and degradation of acetylcholine receptors in rat skeletal muscles. Effects of electrical stimulation. Neuroscience 4:527–538

Lindstrøm J (1983) Acetylcholine receptors: structure, function, synthesis, destruction and antigenicity. In: Engel A, Banker B (eds) Myology, chapter 27. McGraw-Hill, New York

Lindstrøm J, Walter B, Einarson B (1979a) Immunochemical similarities between subunits of acetylcholine receptors from *Torpedo, Electrophorus,* and mammalian muscle. Biochemistry 18:4470–4480

Lindstrøm J, Merlie J, Yogeeswaran G (1979b) Biochemical properties of acetylcholine receptor subunits from *Torpedo californica.* Biochemistry 18:4465–4470

Lo MMS, Garland PB, Lamprecht I, Barnard EA (1980) Rotational mobility of the membrane-bound acetylcholine receptor of *Torpedo* electric organ measured by phosphorescence depolarization. FEBS Lett 111:407–410

Lo MMS, Dolly JO, Barnard EA (1981) Molecular forms of the acetylcholine receptors from vertebrate muscles and *Torpedo* electric organ. Eur J Biochem 116:155–163

Lømo T, Rosenthal J (1972) Control of ACh sensitivity by muscle activity in the rat. J Physiol (Lond) 221:493–513

Lømo T, Westgaard RH (1975) Further studies on the control of ACh sensitivity by muscle activity in the rat. J Physiol (Lond) 252:603–626

Loring RH, Salpeter MM (1980) Denervation increases turnover rate of junctional acetylcholine receptors. Proc Natl Acad Sci USA 77:2293–2297

Maelicke A, Prinz H (1983) The acetylcholine receptor-ion channel complex: linkage between binding and response. In: Satir BH (ed) Modern cell biology, vol 1. Liss, New York, pp 171–197

Magazanik LG, Vyskočil F (1970) Dependence of acetylcholine desensitization on the membrane potential of frog muscle fibre on the ionic changes in the mesium. J Physiol (Lond) 210:507–518

Magazanik LG, Vyskočil F (1973) Desensitization at the motor end-plate. In: Rang HP (ed) Drug receptors. MacMillan, London, pp 105–119

Magazanik LG, Vyskočil F (1975) The effect of temperature on desensitization kinetics at the postsynaptic membrane of the frog muscle fibre. J Physiol Lond 249:285–300

Magazanik LG, Vyskočil F (1976) Desensitization at the neuromuscular junction. In: Thesleff S (ed) Motor innervation of muscle. Academic, London, pp 151–176

Magazanik LG, Nikolsky E, Vyskočil F (1982) Effect of the desensitization-potentiating agent SKF-525A on frog end-plate currents. Eur J Pharmacol 80:115–119

Magleby KL, Pallotta BS (1981) A study of desensitization of acetylcholine receptors using nerve-released transmitter in the frog. J Physiol (Lond) 316:225–250

Magleby KL, Stevens CF (1972) A quantitative description of end-plate currents. J Physiol (Lond) 223:173–197

McArdle JJ (1983) Molecular aspects of the trophic influence of nerve on muscle. Prog Neurobiol 21:135–198

McNamee MG, Ochoa ELM (1982) Reconstitution of acetylcholine receptor function in model membranes. Neuroscience 7:2305–2319

Messing A (1982) Cholinergic agonist down regulation of neuronal alphabungarotoxin receptors. Brain Res 232:479–484

Michler A, Sakmann B (1980) Receptor stability and channel conversion in the subsynaptic membrane of the developing mammalian neuromuscular junction. Dev Biol 80:1–17

Nathanson NM, Hall ZW (1979) Subunit structure and peptide mapping of junctional and extrajunctional acetylcholine receptors from rat muscle. Biochemistry 18:3392–3401

Neher E, Sakmann B (1976a) Noise analysis of drug induced voltage clamp currents in denervated frog muscle fibres. J Physiol (Lond) 258:705–729

Neher E, Sakmann B (1976b) Single-channel currents recorded from membrane of denervated frog muscle fibres. Nature 260:799–802

Nitkin RM, Wallace BG, Spira ME, Godfrey EW, McMahan UJ (1983) Molecular components of the synaptic basal lamina that direct differentiation of regenerating neuromuscular junctions. In: Cold spring harbor symposia on quantitative biology, vol 48. Molecular Neurobiology. Cold Spring Harbor, New York, p 653

Pagala MKD, Namba T, Grob D (1981) Desensitization to acetylcholine at motor end-plates in normal humans, patients with myasthenia gravis and experimental models of myasthenia gravis. Ann NY Acad Sci 377:567–582

Pagala MKD, Tada S, Namba T, Grob D (1982) Neuromuscular transmission in neonatal mice injected with serum globulin of myasthenia gravis patients. Neurology 32:12–17

Peper K, Bradley RJ, Dreyer F (1982) The acetylcholine receptor at the neuromuscular junction. Physiol Rev 62:1271–1340

Polak RL, Sellin LC, Thesleff S (1981) Acetylcholine content and release in denervated or botulinum poisoned rat skeletal muscle. J Physiol (Lond) 319:253–259

Popot JL (1983) Structural and functional properties of the acetylcholine receptor: studies using reconstituted vesicles. In: Jasper HH, van Gelder NM (eds) Basic mechanism of neuronal hyperexcitability. Liss, New York, pp 137–170

Popot JL, Changeux JP (1984) Nicotinic receptor of acetylcholine: Structure of an oligomeric integral membrane protein. Physiol Rev 64:(4)1162–1239

Porter CW, Chiu TH, Wieckowski J, Barnard EA (1973) Types and locations of cholinergic receptor-like molecules in muscle fibres. Nature 241:3–7

Powell JA, Friedman BA (1977) Electrical membrane activity: effect on distribution, incorporation and degradation of acetylcholine receptors in the membranes of cultured muscle. J Cell Biol 75:MU433

Purves D, Sakmann B (1974) The effect of contractile activity on fibrillation and extrajunctional acetylcholine-sensitivity in rat muscle maintained in organ culture. J Physiol (Lond) 237:157–182

Raftery MA, Hunkapiller MW, Strader CD, Hood LE (1980) Acetylcholine receptor: complex of homologous subunits. Science 208:1454–1457

Reynolds JA, Karlin A (1978) Molecular weight in detergent solution of acetylcholine receptor from *Torpedo californica.* Biochemistry 17:2035–2038

Sakmann B, Brenner HR (1978) Change in synaptic channel gating during neuromuscular development. Nature 276:401–402

Sakmann B, Neher E (eds) (1983) Single-channel recording. Plenum, New York

Sakmann B, Patlak J, Neher E (1980) Single acetylcholine-activated channels show burst-kinetics in presence of desensitizing concentrations of agonist. Nature 286:71–73

Sarvey JM, Albuquerque EX, Eldefrawi AT, Eldefrawi M (1978) Effects of alpha-bungarotoxin and reversible cholinergic ligands on normal and denervated mammalian skeletal muscle. Membr Biochem 1:131–157

Schuetze SM, Fischbach GD (1978) Channel open time decreases postnatally in rat synaptic acetylcholine receptors. Soc Neurosci Abs 8:1195

Scubon-Mulieri B, Parsons RL (1978) Desensitization onset and recovery at the potassium-depolarized frog neuromuscular junction are voltage-sensitive. J Gen Physiol 71:285–299

Spivak CE, Albuquerque EX (1982) Dynamic properties of the nicotinic receptor ionic channel complex: activation and blockade. In: Hanin I, Goldberg A (eds) Progress in cholinergic biology: models of cholinergic synapses. Raven, New York, pp 323–357

Stanley EF, Drachman DE (1981) Denervation accelerates the degradation of junctional acetylcholine receptors. Exp Neurol 73:390–396

Steinbach JH (1974) Role of muscle activity in nerve-muscle interaction in vitro. Nature 248:70–71

Stevens CF (1985) AChR structure: a new twist in the story. Trends Neurosci 8:1–2

Stroud RM (1983) Acetylcholine receptor structure. Neurosci Comment 1:124–138

Sun YA, Poo MM (1985) Non-quantal release of acetylcholine at a developing neuromuscular synapse in culture. J Neurosci 5:634–642

Takai T, Noda M, Mishina M, Shimizu S, Furutani Y, Kayano T, Ikeda T, Kubo T, Takahashi H, Takahashi T, Kuno M, Numa S (1985) Cloning, sequensing and expression of cDNA for a novel subunit of acetylcholine receptor from calf muscle. Nature 315:761–764

Taylor P, Sine SM (1981) The relationship between ligand occupation and activation of the nicotinic cholinergic receptor. In: Stjärne L, Hedgvist P, Lagercrantz H, Wennmalem A (eds) Chemical neurotransmission. Seventy-five years. Academic, London, pp 347–359

Taylor JE, Yaksh TL, Richelson E (1982) Agonist regulation of muscarinic acetylcholine receptors in rat spinal cord. J Neurochem 39:521–524

Teichberg VI, Changeux JP (1976) Presence of two forms of acetylcholine receptor with different isoelectric points in the electric organ of *Electrophorus electricus* and their catalytic interconversion in vitro. FEBS Lett 67:264–268

Thesleff S (1955) The mode of neuromuscular block caused by acetylcholine, nicotine, decamethonium and succinylcholine. Acta Physiol Scand 34:218–231

Thesleff S (1959) Motor end-plate "desensitization" by repetitive nerve stimuli. J Physiol (Lond) 148:659–664

Thesleff S, Sellin LC (1980) Denervation supersensitivity. Trends Neurosci 3:122–126

Thoenen H, Korsching S, Barde YA, Edgar D (1983) Quantitation and purification of neurotrophic molecules. In: Cold Spring Harbor Laboratory (eds) Cold Spring Harbor symposia on quantit biol. Mol Neurobiol 48:679

Trautmann A (1982) Curare can open and block ionic channels associated with cholinergic receptors. Nature 298:272–275

Vincent A (1980) Immunology of acetylcholine receptors in relation to myasthenia gravis. Physiol Rev 60:756–824

Vizi ES, Vyskočil F (1979) Changes in total and quantal release of acetylcholine in the mouse diaphragm during activation and inhibition of membrane ATPase. J Physiol (Lond) 286:1–14

Vyskočil F (1974) Action potentials of the rat diaphragm and their sensitivity to tetrodotoxin during postnatal development and old age. Pflugers Arch 352:155–163

Vyskočil F (1975) Recovery of sensitivity to acetylcholine following desensitization in muscles of different vertebrate species. Pflugers Arch 361:83–87

Vyskočil F (1978) Effect of diazepam on the frog neuromuscular junction. Eur J Pharmacol 48:117–124

Vyskočil F, Gutmann E (1976) Control of ACh sensitivity in temporarily unconnected ("decentralized") segments of diaphragm-muscle fibres of the rat. Pflugers Arch 367:43–47

Vyskočil F, Illés P (1977) Non-quantal release of transmitter at mouse neuromuscular junction and its dependence of the activity of Na^{+}-K^{+} ATPase. Pflugers Arch 370:295–297

Vyskočil F, Illés P (1978) Electrophysiological examination of transmitter release in non-quantal form in the mouse diaphragm and the activity of membrane ATPase. Physiol Bohemoslov 27:449–455

Vyskočil F, Syrový I, Prusík Z (1981) Induction of extrajunctional acetylcholine sensitivity of rat EDL muscle by peptidic component of peripheral nerve. Pflugers Arch 390:265–269

Vyskočil F, Nikolsky E, Edwards C (1983) An analysis of the mechanisms underlying the non-quantal release of acetylcholine at the mouse neuromuscular junction. Neuroscience 9(2):429–435

Wennogle LP (1985) The end-plate acetylcholine receptor: structure and function. In: Kharkevich DA (ed) New curare-like agents. Springer, Berlin Heidelberg New York Tokyo (Handbook of experimental pharmacology, vol 79)

Factors Influencing Motor Nerve Growth

C. E. Henderson[1]

Introduction

By far the best-characterized factor affecting nerve growth is the nerve growth factor (NGF), identified in 1956 by Cohen and Levi-Montalcini (for review, see Thoenen and Barde 1980), and subsequently sequenced and cloned. The purified protein has three major effects on sympathetic and sensory neurons cultured at appropriate development stages: it is required for cell survival, and enhances neurite outgrowth and neurotransmitter synthesis.

It is likely that NGF is released by target tissues in order to assure themselves of sufficient sympathetic and sensory innervation. This hypothesis is supported by the observations that: (a) administration of anti-NGF antibodies in newborn mice results in a selective loss of sympathetic neurons, known as "immunosympathectomy" (Levi-Montalcini and Booker 1960); (b) axons of responsive neurons are capable of transporting NGF in a retrograde manner from the nerve terminal to the cell body (Hendry 1976); and (c) levels of NGF in target organs correlate with the density of sympathetic innervation (Korsching and Thoenen 1983).

The characterization of putative nerve growth factors in other parts of the nervous system is considerably less advanced. I will discuss here the evidence that comparable factors play a role in the development and maintenance of the neuromuscular junction, and consider the effects of muscle activity on their production.

Evidence in vivo for the Existence of Muscle-Derived Motoneuron Growth Factors

The first evidence for a dependence of spinal motoneurons on their muscle target came from the classic work of Hamburger (1958). In the lumbar spinal cord of the chick embryo, approximately 50% of the motoneurons initially generated die during the period of "naturally occurring cell death," between embryonic days 5 and 9. Extirpation of a limb bud at an earlier stage (ED3) of development results in the death of 100% of the motoneurons on the operated side, without affecting the contralateral anterior horn. On the other hand, implantation of a supernumerary limb (Hollyday and Hamburger 1976) allows the "rescue" of some of the motoneurons that would normally have died. These results, and others, gave rise to the hypothesis that developing muscle produces limited quantities of a growth factor upon which embryonic motoneurons depend for their survival. Only those successful in "competition"

1 Neurobiologie Moléculaire, Institut Pasteur, 25 rue du Dr. Roux, 75015 Paris, France

Electrical Stimulation and Neuromuscular Disorders
Ed. by W. A. Nix and G. Vrbová

at the periphery for a supply of the factor will survive, and this number can be modulated experimentally by altering the volume of available target tissue.

In other experiments, Lewis et al. (1981) X-irradiated the somites of 2-day embryos so as to generate embryos in which one wing was completely normal and the other was morphologically normal but lacked muscle. Although the principal nerve tracts developed normally in the irradiated wings, specific muscle nerve branches were absent. One interpretation of these results is that the last stages of axon outgrowth also require a muscle-derived factor.

Growth factors have also been implicated at later stages in the process of sprouting of axons in a partially denervated muscle (Brown et al. 1981). The "sprouting signal" is released by denervated muscle fibres and can diffuse a limited distance within the muscle.

Characterization of Putative Motoneuron Growth Factors

The most frequent approach to characterizing the motoneuron growth factors supposed to exist from the above in vivo evidence has been to culture spinal neurons or motoneurons in vitro and to demonstrate an effect of muscle-derived substances on a parameter of neuronal differentiation or survival. Neurons used have ranged from explants of spinal cord (Driblin and Barrett 1982) and dissociated spinal neurons (Tanaka and Obata 1982) to identified (Bennett et al. 1980) or purified (Calof and Reichardt 1984) motoneurons, and factors have been studied affecting their survival (Longo et al. 1982), neurite outgrowth (Pollack et al. 1981) and neurotransmitter synthesis (Giller et al. 1977). No putative motoneuron growth factor has yet been isolated by such methods, and it is thus too early to compare the molecules responsible.

We have used serum-free cultures of dissociated embryonic (4.5 days in ovo) chick spinal neurons to detect and study factors affecting neurite outgrowth (Henderson 1983; Henderson et al. 1981, 1983). Spinal cords were dissected at this early stage with the aim of enriching motoneurons in the cultures, but there is at present no direct evidence that the responsive cells are indeed cholinergic. Neurite-promoting activity was first detected in media conditioned by embryonic myotubes in vitro. The active factor(s) was associated with species of molecular weight 40000 and greater, was trypsin-sensitive and was produced at significant levels only by muscle and liver cells in culture.

Activity was also found in soluble extracts of postnatal chick leg muscle; the levels of this "neonatal" activity increased 10-fold from hatching up to a peak at 3–4 days post-natal, subsequently falling back to basal levels (Henderson et al. 1984). It is tempting to hypothesize that this peak of activity may correspond to the period of synapse elimination in these muscles.

A novel approach to the problem of identifiying motoneuron growth factors has been that of Gurney and collaborators (Gurney 1984; Gurney and Apatoff 1984). They showed that antisera raised against a medium conditioned by denervated skeletal muscle were capable of inhibiting the degree of sprouting in mouse muscle treated with botulinum toxin. The inhibitory population of immunoglobulins recognized a protein of molecular weight 56000. This protein had a survival-promoting activity for embryonic spinal neurons in vitro. Analysis of the effects in vivo of monospecific antibodies directed against the 56 K protein should provide an indication of its biological role.

Growth cones of spinal neurons in vitro will turn and grow towards a source of muscle-conditioned medium released from a micropipette (Gundersen and Park 1984). Media conditioned by other cell types had no effect on directional growth. The same spinal neurons showed selective adhesion to culture substratum pretreated with medium conditioned by muscle, but not other, cells.

In addition to the activities described above, one molecule (or group of molecules) has been shown to have a marked effect on neurite outgrowth from spinal neurons and many other neuronal types (Longo et al. 1982; Lander et al. 1982). Such factors, only active once bound to the culture substratum in vitro, have a molecular structure similar to that of laminin, to which they show, after denaturation by SDS, limited antigenic cross-reactivity. They are produced by almost all cell types in culture and thus, while probably playing an important role in cell-cell interactions, do not fulfil the criteria for identification of the hypothetical motoneuron growth factor.

Effects of Activity on Growth Factor Production

Among the target tissues known to produce NGF is the rat iris (Korsching and Thoenen 1983). Ebendal et al. (1980) showed that levels of NGF (assayed by its effect on embryonic ganglia in vitro) were increased by at least one order of magnitude 10 days after sensory or sympathetic denervation but fell back to barely detectable levels concomitant with reinnervation of iris grafts. Although part of this increase may be due to interruption of retrograde transport of NGF by the sensory and sympathetic axons, there is a marked effect on de novo synthesis, as shown by measuring levels of specific mRNA (Shelton and Reichardt 1984).

At the neuromuscular junction, several experiments in vivo suggest that an active muscle produces less of the hypothetical motoneuron growth factor than does an inactive muscle. Sprouting in partially denervated adult muscle is completely suppressed by direct stimulation of the muscle (Brown and Holland 1979). If, at early embryonic stages, cholinergic transmission is blocked by administration of curare, the number of motoneurons surviving the period of naturally-occurring cell death is increased to virtually 100% (Pittman and Oppenheim 1978), whereas direct stimulation during this period accentuates cell death.

In an attempt to observe an effect of muscle activity using our in vitro bioassay, we denervated muscles of 6-day post-hatch chicks by section of the sciatic nerve under anaesthesia (Henderson et al. 1983). Three days later, extracts were prepared from the denervated muscles and from control muscles in the contralateral leg, sham-operated chicks and non-operated chicks. The extracts were assayed for their activity in promoting neurite outgrowth. The specific activity of the denervated muscle extracts was 10- to 15-fold greater than that of the controls, and the time course of appearance of the denervation effect (3 days) was comparable to the period (4–6 days) that elapses in partially denervated mammalian muscle before the first sprouts are detected. Similar results have been reported for survival-promoting activities (Slack and Pockett 1982; Hill and Bennett 1983).

The striking effect of denervation could have been the result of the interruption of muscle contractile activity, or could be caused by nerve degeneration products. We have measured neurite-promoting activities in two other experimental systems in which activity is lowered but in which there is no surgical intervention on the nerve: the *paralysé* mouse mutant and tenotomised muscle of neonatal rat. In each case, there was a significant increase in specific activity (Henderson et al. 1986). However, until direct stimulation of the affected muscles has been performed, it will not be certain that these effects result from activity changes.

Relevance to Electrical Stimulation in the Clinical Context

It is clear that our knowledge of the putative motoneuron growth factors is extremely limited, and such results as there are must be extrapolated with the utmost caution to the clinical context. Apart from the fact that the molecules involved remain for the most part uncharacterized, and totally so in man, their role in vivo has in no case been demonstrated. In addition, the spinal motoneuron has an extremely complex cellular environment, both centrally and peripherally, and the putative muscle-derived factors are probably not the only trophic influence to which the motoneuron is subject.

One point, however, perhaps deserves attention. It is clear from the effect of direct stimulation on sprouting (Brown and Holland 1979), and suggested by other in vivo and in vitro results discussed above (Henderson et al. 1983; Slack and Pockett 1982; Hill and Bennett 1983), that inactive muscle produces more growth-promoting factors than does active muscle. This fits well with the idea that the role of such factors is to ensure that the target muscle is sufficiently innervated (or re-innervated following injury). It is thus conceivable that electrical stimulation used clinically might slow down processes of reinnervation (but see Nix 1982, 1986). Such simplistic arguments do not take into account the complexity of the system, for instance the necessity for maintaining muscle survival during reinnervation. It is to be hoped that carefully controlled studies of the effects of electrical stimulation in animal models, combined with further characterization of the molecules affecting motor nerve growth, will allow a more systematic approach to the clinical problem.

Acknowledgements. I wish to thank my collaborators M. Huchet, P. Benoît, J. L. Guénet, H. Nuret and J. P. Changeux who participated in the studies described in this article.

References

Bennett MR, Lai K, Nurcombe V (1980) Identification of embryonic motoneurons in vitro: their survival is dependent on skeletal muscle. Brain Res 190:537–542

Brown MC, Holland RL (1979) A central role for denervated tissues in causing nerve sprouting. Nature 282:724–726

Brown MC, Holland RL, Hopkins WG (1981) Motor nerve sprouting. Annu Rev Neurosci 4:17–42

Calof AL, Reichardt LF (1984) Motoneurons purified by cell sorting respond to two distinct activities in myotube-conditioned medium. Dev Biol 106:194–210

Dribin LB, Barrett JN (1982) Two components of conditioned medium increase neuritic outgrowth from rat spinal cord explants. J Neurosci Res 8:271–280

Ebendal T, Olson L, Seiger A, Hedlund KO (1980) Nerve growth factors in the rat iris. Nature 286:25–28

Giller EL, Neale JH, Bullock PN, Schrier BK, Nelson PG (1977) Choline acetyltransferase activity of spinal cord cell cultures increased by co-culture with muscle and by muscle-conditioned medium. J Cell Biol 74:16–29

Gundersen RW, Park KHC (1984) The effects of conditioned media on spinal neurites: substrate-associated changes in neurite direction and adherence. Dev Biol 104:18–27

Gurney ME (1984) Suppression of terminal sprouting at the neuromuscular junction by immune sera. Nature 307:546–548

Gurney ME, Apatoff B (1984) Activity of a muscle-derived growth factor for spinal neurons in vitro and in vivo. Soc Neurosci Abstr 10:1051

Hamburger V (1958) Regression versus peripheral control of differentiation in motor hypoplasia. Am J Anat 102:365–410

Henderson CE (1983) Roles for retrograde factors in synapse formation at the nerve-muscle junction. Prog Brain Res 58:369–373

Henderson CE, Huchet M, Changeux JP (1981) Neurite outgrowth from embryonic spinal neurons is promoted by media conditioned by muscle cells. Proc Natl Acad Sci USA 78:2625–2629

Henderson CE, Huchet M, Changeux JP (1983) Denervation increases a neurite-promoting activity in extracts of skeletal muscle. Nature 302:609–611

Henderson CE, Huchet M, Changeux JP (1984) Neurite-promoting activities for embryonic spinal neurons and their developmental changes in the chick. Dev Biol 104:336–347

Henderson CE, Benoit P, Huchet M, Guénet JL, Changeux JP (1986) Increase of neurite-promoting activity for spinal neurons in muscles of "paralysé" mice and tenotomised rats. Dev Brain Res 25:65–70

Hendry IA (1976) Control in the development of the vertebrate sympathetic nervous system. Rev Neurosci 2:149–194

Hill MA, Bennett MR (1983) Cholinergic growth factor from skeletal muscle elevated following denervation. Neurosci Lett 35:31–35

Hollyday M, Hamburger V (1976) Reduction of the naturally occurring motor neuron loss by enlargement of the periphery. J Comp Neurol 170:311–320

Korsching S, Thoenen H (1983) Nerve growth factor in sympathetic ganglia and corresponding target organs of the rat: correlation with density of sympathetic innervation. Proc Natl Acad Sci USA 80:3513–3516

Lander AD, Fujii D, Gospadorowicz D, Reichardt LF (1982) Characterization of a factor that promotes neurite outgrowth: evidence linking activity to a heparan sulfate proteoglycan. J Cell Biol 94:574–585

Levi-Montalcini R, Booker B (1960) Destruction of the sympathetic ganglia in mammals by an antiserum to the nerve-growth promoting factor. Proc Natl Acad Sci USA 42:384–391

Lewis J, Chevallier A, Kieny M, Wolpert L (1981) Muscle nerve branches do not develop in chick wings devoid of muscle. J Embryol Exp Morphol 64:211–232

Longo FM, Manthorpe M, Varon S (1982) Spinal cord neuronotrophic factors. I. Bioassay of schwannoma and other conditioned media. Dev Brain Res 3:277–294

Nix WA (1982) The effect of low-frequency electrical stimulation on the denervated extensor digitorum longus muscle of the rabbit. Acta Neurol Scand 66:521–528

Nix WA (1986) Maintenance of muscle integrity following denervation. In: Dimitrijevic M, Kakulas BA, Vrbová G (eds) Recent achievements in restorative neurology. vol 3. Karger, Basel (in press)

Pittman RH, Oppenheim RW (1978) Neuromuscular blockade increase motoneurone survival during normal cell death in the chick embryo. Nature 271:364–366

Pollack ED, Muhlach WL, Liebig V (1981) Neurotropic influence of mesenchymal limb target tissue on spinal cord neurite growth in vitro. J Comp Neurol 177:87–112

Shelton DL, Reichardt LF (1984) Expression of the β-NGF gene correlates with the density of sympathetic innervation in effector organs. Proc Natl Acad Sci USA 81:7951–7955

Slack JR, Pockett S (1982) Motor neurotrophic factor in denervated adult skeletal muscle. Brain Res 247:138–140

Tanaka H, Obata K (1982) Survival and neurite outgrowth of chick embryo spinal cord cells in serum-free culture. Dev Brain Res 4:313–321

Thoenen H, Barde Y-A (1980) Physiology of nerve growth factor. Physiol Rev 60:1284–1335

II. Repair Processes in the Peripheral Nervous System

Neural Activity and the Reorganization of Motor Units in Reinnervated Skeletal Muscle*

R. R. Ribchester[1]

Introduction

The control of voluntary muscle contraction rests ultimately in the 'final common path' – the spinal motoneurons and the muscle fibres they innervate (Sherrington 1906). Peripheral nerve injury requires compensation for the loss of muscle innervation, if the quality of muscle control is to be restored. Compensation in the motor system may occur at many levels: peripheral, spinal and supraspinal (Tsukuhara 1981). In the periphery, denervation of skeletal muscle fibres provokes two mechanisms: sprouting, from intact motor axon collaterals and their terminals; and regeneration of the injured axons (Brown et al. 1981). Sprouting provides a relatively rapid and effective restoration of muscle function, but it is unsatisfactory because the sprouted motor units are expanded. Fine motor control is therefore further compromised.

Regeneration of damaged motor axons does not necessarily redress the balance. A number of studies have shown that regenerating motor axons fail to reinnervate muscle fibres in the numbers they innervated before injury, especially if the target muscle is completely reinnervated by sprouts from intact motor innervation (Brown and Ironton 1978; Thompson 1978). This failure may be attributed partly to the occupancy of motor end-plates by sprouts. Evidently, regenerating axons vie with intact axons for synaptic space. A clearer understanding of the cellular mechanisms of such competition may indicate ways in which the motor system might be manipulated during peripheral nerve regeneration; ways which might facilitate the recovery of precise motor control.

Motoneurons differ in the patterns of nerve impulse activity they express (Hennig and Lømo 1985), and there is evidence that activity can affect the size of motor units. For example it is well established that paralysis of skeletal muscles, produced by blocking nerve impulse conduction or synaptic transmission with neurotoxins, leads to motor nerve sprouting (Brown and Ironton 1977; Duchen 1970; Holland and Brown 1980). During postnatal development of motor units, paralysis inhibits motor unit reorganization, and stimulation accelerates it (Benoit and Changeux 1975; Brown et al. 1982; Caldwell and Ridge 1983; Duxson 1982; O'Brien et al. 1978; Ridge and Betz 1984; Thompson et al. 1979; Thompson 1983). Paralysis also inhibits or prevents elimination of polyneuronal innervation of muscle fibres in reinnervated adult skeletal muscle (Benoit and Changeux 1978; Taxt 1983b).

* This work was supported by the Medical Research Council and Action Research – The National Fund for Research into Crippling Diseases

1 Department of Physiology, University Medical School, Teviot Place, Edinburgh, EH8 9AG, Scotland

Electrical Stimulation and Neuromuscular Disorders
Ed. by W. A. Nix and G. Vrbová

However, there is also evidence that the size of a motor unit depends on intrinsic, metabolic properties of the cells. Motoneurons with large somata and axons normally innervate more muscle fibres than small motoneurons (Henneman et al. 1965; Brown and Ironton 1978; Burke et al. 1982). Furthermore, the extent of motor axon sprouting after partial denervation appears limited, so that only about five times the original complement of muscle fibres can be captured by sprouts (Brown and Ironton 1978; Thompson and Jansen 1977). When a foreign nerve is implanted into a denervated skeletal muscle, the distribution of motor unit sizes is characteristic of the nerve implant, rather than of the muscle implanted (Taxt 1983a). It therefore becomes important to establish to what extent the distribution of motor unit sizes depends on their relative activity patterns, and to what extent it depends on their intrinsic, metabolic properties.

The present paper reviews briefly our recent evidence that differences in the activity of regenerating motor axons influence the number of muscle fibres they ultimately innervate (Betz et al. 1980b; Ribchester and Taxt 1983, 1984). Additional evidence is presented which suggests that activity is the main, but by no means exclusive, determinant of the outcome of neuromuscular synapse elimination during muscle reinnervation.

Experimental Procedures

All the experiments were performed on adult rat lumbrical muscles. The fourth deep lumbrical muscle in the hind foot receives its motor innervation from the lateral plantar nerve (LPN) and a branch of the sural nerve (SN), which fuses with LPN near the ankle. (This functional anatomy is also found in mice and hamsters, but not in rabbits or cats; nor of course in man, where the sural nerve is purely sensory.) Because the LPN and SN are anatomically distinct, the motor axons innervating the lumbrical muscle can be manipulated independently. Motor unit recordings show that this muscle, which contains about 1000 muscle fibres, is innervated by 9–14 motor axons. Most of the motor axons are supplied by the lateral plantar nerve. Up to six may reach the muscle via the sural nerve, but in most animals the SN contains only one to three motor axons (Betz et al. 1979, 1980a).

This unique distribution of the motor axons permits an approach to four separate but related questions. First, what is the role of neuronal activity in the sprouting of intact motor axons? Second, does an active motor nerve terminal have a competitive advantage over an inactive terminal when both converge on a single muscle fibre? Third, can active motor axons repress and displace established but inactive terminals on paralysed muscle fibres? Finally, can muscle fibres reinnervated by functional, collateral sprouts sustain their innervation when inactive motor axons return?

These questions were addressed by studying the properties of motor units in lumbrical muscles in which nerve impulse conduction in the LPN motor axons was blocked. To address the first, innervated muscles were studied. For the second, muscles were completely denervated and the LPN was blocked during nerve regeneration. In the third and fourth, partially denervated muscles were studied. The LPN

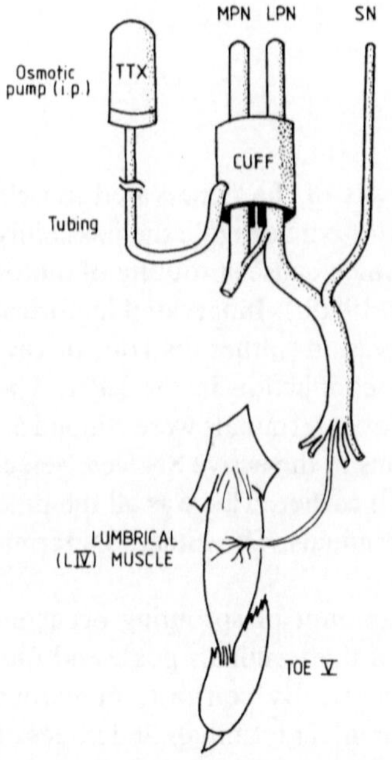

Fig. 1. Schematic diagram of the fourth deep lumbrical muscle and its innervation by branches of the sural nerve *(SN)* and the lateral plantar nerve *(LPN)*. The LPN runs adjacent to the medial plantar nerve *(MPN)* in the shank. Also shown schematically is the method for producing chronic nerve conduction block in the LPN. Silicon rubber tubing interconnects an osmotic minipump (Alzet 2002; 0.5 µl/h) containing dissolved tetrodotoxin (*TTX;* 500 µg/ml), and a loose-fitting silicone rubber cuff. The tubing opens into the lumen of the cuff, which serves a dual purpose: to keep the source of TTX as close to the nerve as possible and to restrict diffusion of the toxin. This procedure was used in conjunction with either muscle nerve crush, SN crush, or LPN crush

was blocked either during the regeneration of SN motor axons only, or during regeneration of LPN motor axons.

Most of the methods have been described in detail elsewhere (Ribchester and Taxt 1983). Briefly, partial or complete denervation of the lumbrical muscles was produced by crushing the muscle nerve (complete denervation), the SN (minor partial denervation) or the LPN (major partial denervation). In addition, complete nerve conduction block in the LPN was accomplished by treating the nerve with tetrodotoxin (Fig. 1). This toxin does not inhibit axonal transport (Bray et al. 1979) and can be used to dissociate the effects of neuromuscular activity from other factors that depend on the structural integrity of neuromuscular synapses. On the day of the acute experiment, the animals were anaesthetized with Sagatal (80 mg/kg) and nerve block was confirmed by stimulating electrically above the LPN cuff or below it, while observing muscle contractions in the foot. Muscle tension responses and intracellular recordings were registered in isolated preparations, dissected with the LPN and SN intact. For tension measurements, the proximal tendon was attached to a sensitive force transducer (AE 801, Akers Engineering, Norway). The fifth toe, with the attached distal tendon, was pinned to the base of a Sylgard-lined chamber. The preparation was superfused at room temperature with oxygenated mammalian saline, pH 7.2 (Liley 1956). For intracellular recordings, cut muscle fibre preparations were used to abolish muscle action potentials. Endplate potentials were recorded using glass microelectrodes filled with 4 *M* potassium acetate.

Review of Findings

Innervated Muscles

The immediate effect of partial denervation is paralysis of the denervated muscle fibres. The purpose of the first group of experiments was to investigate the possibility that inactivity of muscle fibres initiates mechanisms which cause sprouting of motor axons on normal, innervated muscle fibres (Betz et al. 1980b). Innervated lumbrical muscles were subjected to a "functional" partial denervation (rather than one involving nerve degeneration), by blocking nerve impulse conduction in the LPN. The properties of motor units and the structure of motor nerve terminals were studied 5–14 days later. Motor nerve terminals belonging to axons in the active SN were selectively visualized by cutting the blocked LPN axons 24 h earlier. This was all the time needed to cause degeneration of the blocked nerve terminals. The intact, SN terminals were then stained with zinc iodide-osmium.

There were two main findings. First, a modest amount of sprouting occurred from the intact, active nerve terminals. About 35% of the terminals possessed fine sprouts, but these extended only about 13 μm at most. By contrast, numerous sprouts extended for more considerable distances from intact terminals and nodes of Ranvier in muscles that were partially denervated for 5 days or more. Secondly, few sprouts in the partially paralyzed muscles extended to adjacent muscle fibres. Intracellular recordings produced no evidence of polyneuronal innervation of muscle fibres, and there was no evidence that the size or function of blocked or active motor units was altered. Again, this was in contrast to muscles that were partially denervated for comparable periods.

The main conclusion from this work was that muscle inactivity provides a small, but significant stimulus to the sprouting of active motor axons. Denervation of the muscle fibres provides additional stimuli, to which the effects of inactivity are additive. Similar conclusions were reached in experiments performed by M. C. Brown and his colleagues (reviewed by Brown et al. 1981). The additional stimuli provided by partial denervation probably have qualitatively different effects on the sprouting of intact axons in addition to the quantitative ones: nodal sprouting occurs from intact axons in partially denervated muscles, but not from active nerve terminals in inactive muscles (see also Keynes et al. 1983).

Reinnervated Muscles

The next series of experiments addressed the role of activity in motor axons during the regeneration of neuromuscular synapses (Ribchester and Taxt 1983). If active motor nerve terminals were to sustain a competitive advantage over inactive terminals when they transiently converge on single muscle fibres (McArdle 1975), then one would expect the active terminals to persist and the inactive terminals to be eliminated selectively. Accordingly, the active motor units would become larger at the expense of inactive motor units. Our investigation suggested that the outcome of such competitive interactions does depend on motoneuron activity, as elsewhere in the nervous system (see Ribchester 1986).

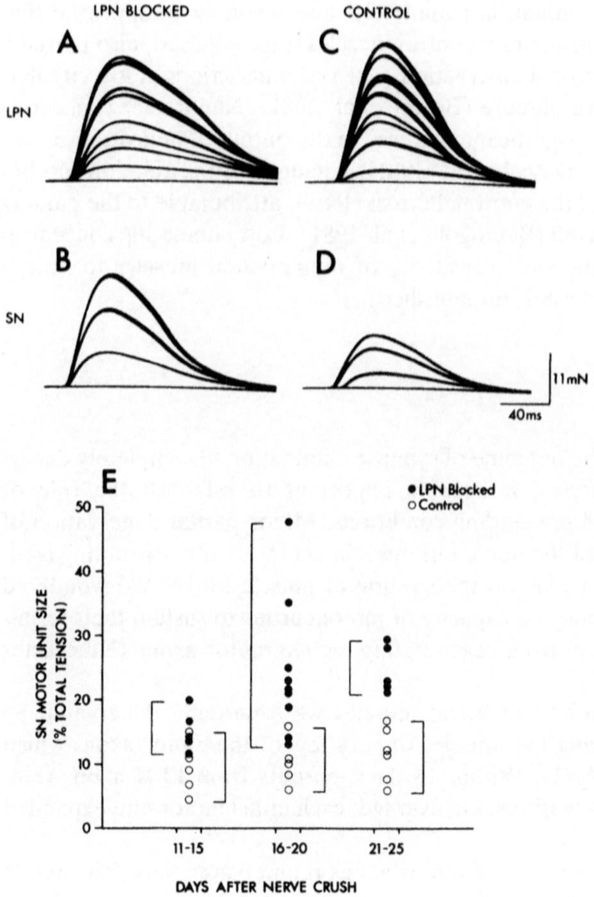

Fig. 2. A–D Motor unit twitch tension recordings from reinnervated lumbrical muscles obtained in an acute experiment, after chronic paralysis of LPN motor units on one side for 10 days. These recordings were taken from a pair of muscles 20 days after crushing the muscle nerve. Stimuli to the LPN and SN were carefully graded in intensity to excite motor axons of successively higher electrical threshold. There were similar numbers of motor units on both sides, but the SN motor units were about twice as large in the LPN-blocked muscle compared with the control. The graph summarizes data on SN motor unit twitch tensions in LPN-blocked *(filled circles)* and control *(open circles)*. By 21–25 days, the SN motor units in LPN blocked muscles were all about twice as large as in controls. (From Ribchester and Taxt 1983)

Adult lumbrical muscles were completely denervated by crushing the muscle nerve. Upon regeneration of the motor axons, conduction in the LPN was blocked with tetrodotoxin (TTX). Muscles were studied by making tension measurements, intracellular recordings and zinc iodide-osmium staining. After 10–14 days of LPN block, motor units innervated by SN motor axons developed about twice as much tension as in control muscles (Fig. 2). There was a concomitant reduction in the tetanic tension generated by the stimulating the LPN motor axons. Zinc iodide-osmium staining confirmed that more muscle fibres were innervated by the active motor axons than normal. Intracellular recordings showed that competition took place at the motor endplates of muscle fibres that were polyneuronally innervated by LPN and SN motor axons. The overall level of polyneuronal innervation of muscle fibres did not change during this period, in spite of the increase in the SN innervation and the decrease in the LPN innervation. This suggests that competition was a continuous process in these muscles, and active motor axons continually retrieved muscle fibres from paralyzed motor units.

Two additional, noteworthy observations were made in the course of this study (Taxt 1983b). First, it was confirmed that complete paralysis of the reinnervated muscles prevented synapse elimination completely; and secondly, it appeared that circulating TTX, to which contralateral control muscles were exposed, also partially sustained the level of polyneuronal innervation. The systemic actions of low circulating concentrations of TTX are obscure (Bower et al. 1981). Nanomolar concentrations of the toxin can produce significant decrease in the output of neurotransmitter from motor nerve terminals (Dascal et al. 1981). Changes in the relationship between membrane proteins and the neuronal cytoskeleton, attributable to the binding of TTX, have also been reported (Baumgold et al. 1981). Low circulating concentrations of TTX also prolong the supersensitivity of reinnervated muscles to acetylcholine (R. Price and R. Ribchester, unpublished).

Minor Partial Denervation

Because activity influenced the outcome of synapse elimination in completely denervated and reinnervated muscles, it became important to establish the role of neuronal activity under more demanding conditions. Minor partial denervation of skeletal muscles leaves most of the nerve terminals intact. Very little sprouting is required to produce complete collateral innervation of muscle fibres. We wondered whether inactivity would impair the capacity of motoneurons to sustain their terminals in the face of competition from regenerating, active motor axons (Ribchester and Taxt 1984).

To test this possibility, adult lumbrical muscles were partially denervated by crushing the SN, thus depriving the muscles of very few of the motor axons which normally innervate them (Fig. 1). Within 16 days, sprouts from LPN axons reinnervated the denervated muscle fibres. On average, each intact motor unit expanded by about 10%.

In control muscles, regenerating SN motor axons reinnervated very few muscle fibres. By 40 days, each SN motor unit comprised only about 2% of the muscle, or about one-fifth the normal proportion. However, when LPN motor axons were blocked, regenerating SN motor units recovered to about normal size (Fig. 3). Unlike the outcome in completely denervated muscles, SN motor axons never reinnervated a larger than normal number of muscle fibres. They were not incapable of doing so; when SN axons alone regenerated into completely denervated muscles, they reinnervated five to ten times the normal number of muscle fibres (Fig. 3d).

These results suggest that regenerating, active motor axons can selectively repress intact, but inactive, motor nerve terminals. Their capacity to do so is limited, however, and other factors are important. One possibility is that these factors may be associated with the capacity of motoneurons to support metabolically only a limited number of terminals. The final group of experiments in this series was designed to investigate this possibility.

Major Partial Denervation

Extensive partial denervation of lumbrical muscles was achieved by crushing the LPN. This procedure left most muscles innervated by between one and three SN

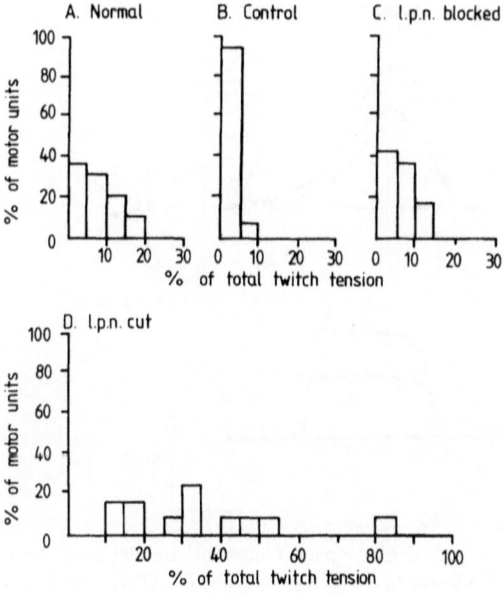

Fig. 3 A–D. Histograms showing the distribution of SN motor units sizes in unoperated muscles (**A**), and muscles in which the LPN was blocked during SN regeneration (**C**); compared with controls in which the LPN was not blocked (**B**) or in which it was cut (**D**). In the LPN-blocked muscles, the distribution of regenerated motor unit sizes is similar to that in unoperated muscles and significantly larger than in controls, but significantly smaller than in muscles innervated only by the SN (From Ribchester and Taxt 1984)

motor axons (Fig. 1). Complete reinnervation of the muscle therefore required extensive sprouting by SN motor axon collaterals. Sprouting of SN terminals following LPN lesions is easily seen using zinc iodide-osmium staining (Betz et al. 1980b) and by the increase in SN motor unit tension. By 16 days, stimulation of the SN produced tension responses that were similar to those obtained by supramaximal, direct muscle stimulation – provided the SN supplied two or more motor units.

Regenerating LPN motor axons returned to the muscles by about 18 days after the initial surgery. Thus, the regenerating motor axons – deprived of their targets – returned to muscles innervated by very few, intact motor axons. The intact motor units were probably as large as the parent motoneurons could support metabolically. In controls, the LPN tension recovered to normal with time in many cases. In some muscles, however, LPN motor axons developed less than half the muscle tension, even 2 months after their return. There was a net decrease in the size of the sprouted, SN motor units in the reinnervated muscles. But again, in some muscles single SN motor axons innervated more than 50% of the muscle up to 2 months after LPN crush (Ribchester 1984). It was as if regenerating LPN axons exuberantly formed new synaptic connections on returning to the lumbrical muscle, but then synapse elimination occured nonselectively between terminals belonging to SN and LPN motor axons.

To test whether motoneuron activity might be important in interactions between expanded SN motor units and exuberant LPN axons, activity in the regenerating motor axons was blocked with TTX from 18–21 days after crushing the LPN. Muscles were studied in acute experiments 9–13 days later, that is, 27–33 days after the original surgery. Tension recordings from an LPN-blocked muscle and its contralateral control are shown in Fig. 4. There were two significant findings. First, the tension responses produced by stimulating the blocked, regenerating axons were about

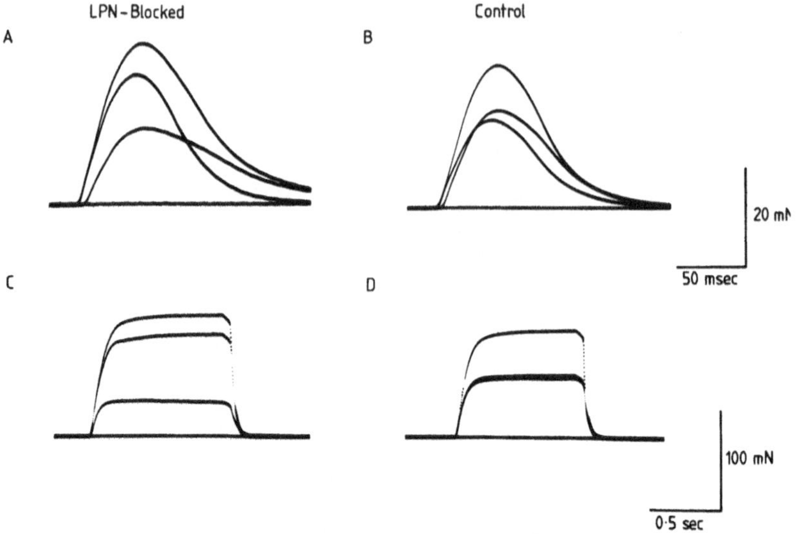

Fig. 4 A–D. Twitch and tetanic muscle tension recordings in a pair of lumbrical muscles made during regeneration of LPN motor axons, 33 days after crushing the LPN. The LPN was blocked for 12 days in the case of the recordings shown on the left (**A, C**). In each case, the smallest tension response was obtained by stimulating the LPN motor axons, the middle trace is the SN tension response and the upper trace combined nerve stimulation. The SN contained three motor axons in both these muscles and the LPN contributed seven and eight motor units respectively. Note the prolonged twitch of the LPN tension in the LPN-blocked muscle. This is a characteristic feature of the paralyzed motor units and is partly due to repetitive firing in the blocked motor axons when they are stimulated electrically (Taxt 1983b). The fused tetanic tension responses (70 Hz) give a more reliable indication of the proportion of muscle fibres innervated by the blocked and active nerves

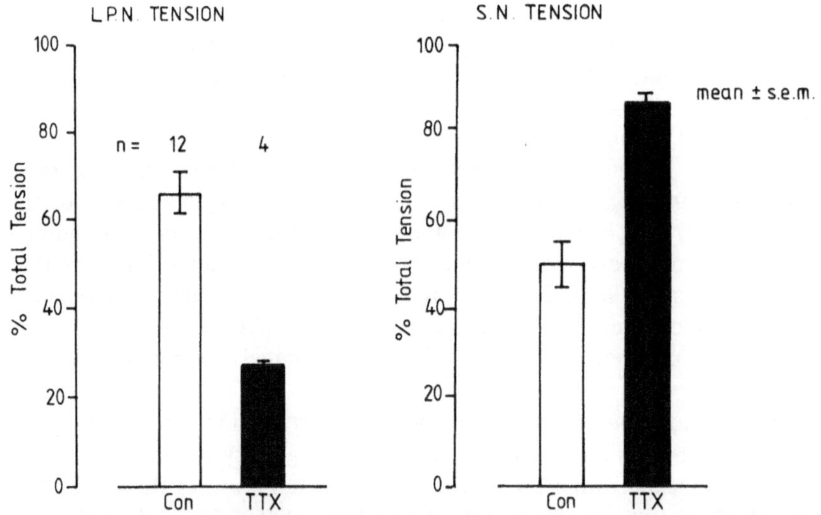

Fig. 5. Comparison of the mean (± SEM) LPN and SN tetanic tension responses in muscles examined between 25–35 days after crushing the LPN. Open bars, control muscles; filled bars, 9–13 days of LPN block. The LPN produced consistently less tension in LPN-blocked muscles than in controls, and the SN tension responses were consistently larger ($P<0.02$; *t*-test)

half that in controls (Fig. 5). This result is consistent with our earlier observations, described in the preceding sections. It indicates that inactivity impairs the capacity of regenerating motor axons to establish or consolidate synaptic connections in completely innervated, active muscles.

The second, and perhaps more surprising finding was that in every muscle, some muscle fibres became exclusively reinnervated by inactive motor axons. There was evidence for this in the tension measurements: combined nerve stimulation always produced more tension than SN stimulation alone (Fig. 4). The mean contribution by fibres innervated by the LPN alone was calculated to be 13.9% ± 2.3% of the total (mean ± SD). Nevertheless, this was significantly less than in contralateral controls (40.1% ± 17.8%). The possibility that the excess tension was due to muscle fibres which retained a subthreshold SN input was ruled out by intracellular recording from muscle fibres (Fig. 6): 31.4% of fibres impaled with microelectrodes produced end-plate potentials to LPN stimulation only ($n = 86$ fibres in three muscles). Thus, it appears that despite their inactivity, the regenerating LPN axons could displace active SN terminals from some muscle fibres. As a result, muscle fibres that were initially active due to their SN innervation became paralyzed due to the substitution of inactive LPN terminals.

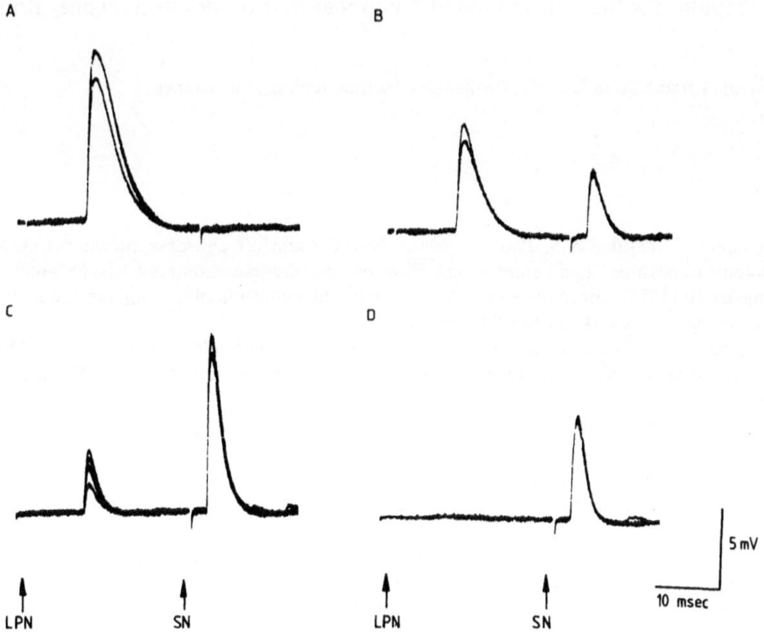

Fig. 6 A–D. End plate potentials recorded in a cut-muscle fibre preparation 28 days after LPN crush. The LPN was blocked from 21 days post crush until the time these recordings were made. In each record, the LPN was stimulated first and the SN about 20 ms later. **A** Muscle fibre innervated only by an LPN motor axon. Note the prolonged repolarization, characteristic of muscle fibres reinnervated by an inactive nerve. **B, C** Dual-innervated fibres, with inputs from LPN and SN motor axons. **D** Muscle fibre innervated only by an SN motor axon

General Conclusions

Disparities in the size of competing motor units and disparities in their activity may both influence the numbers of muscle fibres they ultimately innervate. Neither factor is overriding. This suggests that, at the level of single muscle fibres, interactions involving convergent nerve terminals have a stochastic, unpredictable quality: for a given muscle fibre it may be impossible to say which terminals shall persist and which are to be eliminated.

It should be possible to test this hypothesis. The most productive approach might be to study synapse elimination in culture, where culture conditions or the acitvity of motor axons might more easily be manipulated (Fischman and Nelson 1981; Schaffner et al. 1984). It will be important to develop a protocol in which focal convergence of motoneurons onto single muscle fibres is produced reliably in vitro, and in which it is possible to monitor synapse elimination continuously. It should then be possible to predict the overall pattern of innervation and whether the average probability of persistence or withdrawal of terminals depends mainly on the activity of competing motoneurons.

Finally, the experiments described here may have some implications for the role of activity in the clinical management of peripheral nerve regeneration. In particular, they imply caution in the use of electrical stimulation if the object is to repair neuromuscular function. Our results suggest that *inactivity* in intact motor units is a more potent stimulus for the reformation of functional connections by a regenerating nerve.

Acknowledgements. I thank Julie Douglas for her outstanding technical assistance.

References

Baumgold J, Gallant P, Terekawa S, Paut H (1981) Tetrodotoxin affects submembranous cytoskeletal proteins in perfused squid giant axons. Biochem Biophys Res Commun 103:653–658

Benoit P, Changeux JP (1975) Consequences of tenotomy on the evolution of multiinervation in developing rat soleus muscles. Brain Res 99:354–358

Benoit P, Changeux JP (1978) Consequences of blocking the nerve with a local anaesthetic on the evolution of multiinervation at the regenerating neuromuscular junction of the rat. Brain Res 149:89–96

Betz WJ, Caldwell JH, Ribchester RR (1979) The size of motor units during postnatal development of rat lumbrical muscle. J Physiol (Lond) 297:463–478

Betz WJ, Caldwell JH, Ribchester RR (1980a) The effects of partial denervation at birth on the development of muscle fibres and motor units in rat lumbrical muscles. J Physiol (Lond) 303:265–279

Betz WJ, Caldwell JH, Ribchester RR (1980b) Sprouting of active nerve terminals in partially inactive muscles of the rat. J Physiol (Lond) 303:281–297

Bower DJ, Hart RS, Matthews PA, Howden MEH (1981) Non-protein neurotoxins. Clin Toxicol 18:813–863

Bray JJ, Hubbard JI, Mills RG (1979) The trophic influence of tetrodotoxin-inactive nerves on normal and reinnervated rat skeletal muscles. J Physiol (Lond) 297:479–491

Brown MC, Ironton R (1977) Motor nerve sprouting induced by prolonged tetrodotoxin block of nerve action potentials. Nature 265:459–461

Brown MC, Ironton R (1978) Sprouting and regression of neuromuscular synapses in partially denervated mammalian muscles. J Physiol (Lond) 278:325–348

Brown MC, Holland RL, Hopkins WG (1981) Motor nerve sprouting. Annu Rev Neurosci 4:17–42
Brown MC, Hopkins RL, Keynes RJ (1982) Short- and long-term effects of paralysis on the motor innervation of two different neonatal mouse muscles. J Physiol (Lond) 329:439–450
Burke RE, Dunn RP, Fleshman JW, Glenn LL, Lev-Tov A, O'Donovan MJ, Pinter MJ (1982) An HRP study of the relation between cell size and motor unit type in cat extensor motoneurons. J Comp Neurol 209:17–28
Caldwell JH, Ridge RMAP (1983) The effects of de-afferentation and spinal cord transection on synapse elimination in developing rat muscle. J Physiol (Lond) 339:145–160
Dascal N, Landau EM, Lass Y (1981) Divalent cations and transmitter release at low concentrations of tetrodotoxin. Biophys J 35:573–586
Duchen LW (1970) Changes in motor innervation and cholinesterase localization induced by botulinum toxin in skeletal muscle of the mouse: differences between fast and slow muscles. J Neurol Neurosurg Psychiatry 33:40–54
Duxson MJ (1982) The effect of post-synaptic block on development of the neuromuscular junction in postnatal rats. J Neurocytol 11:395–408
Fischman MC, Nelson PG (1981) Depolarization-induced synaptic plasticity at cholinergic synapses in tissue culture. J Neurosci 1:1043–1051
Henneman E, Somjen G, Olsen DO (1965) Functional significance of cell size in spinal motoneurons. J Neurophysiol 28:560–583
Hennig R, Lømo T (1985) Firing patterns of motor units in normal rats. Nature 314:164–166
Holland RL, Brown MC (1980) Post-synaptic transmission block can cause motor nerve terminal sprouting. Science 207:649–651
Keynes RJ, Hopkins WG, Brown MC (1983) Sprouting of mammalian motoneurones at nodes of Ranvier: the role of the denervated motor endplate. Brain Res 264:209–213
Liley AW (1956) An investigation of spontaneous activity at the neuromuscular junction of the rat. J Physiol (Lond) 132:650–666
McArdle JJ (1975) Complex end-plate potentials at the regenerating neuromuscular junction of the rat. Exp Neurol 49:629–638
O'Brien RAD, Östberg AJC, Vrbová G (1978) Observations on the elimination of polyneuronal innervation in developing mammalian skeletal muscle. J Physiol (Lond) 282:571–582
Ribchester RR (1984) Non-selective elimination of motor nerve terminals after reinnervation of partially denervated rat lumbrical muscle. J Physiol (Lond) 346:25P
Ribchester RR (1986) Molecule, nerve and embryo, chap 6. Blackie, Glasgow
Ribchester RR, Taxt T (1983) Motor unit size and synaptic competition in rat lumbrical muscles reinnervated by active and inactive motor axons. J Physiol (Lond) 344:89–111
Ribchester RR, Taxt T (1984) Repression of inactive motor nerve terminals in partially denervated rat muscle after regeneration of active motor axons. J Physiol (Lond) 347:497–511
Ridge RMAP, Betz WJ (1984) The effect of selective chronic stimulation on motor unit size in developing rat muscle. J Neurosci 4:2614–2620
Schaffner AE, Nelson PG, Fischman MC (1984) Synapse repression in cell culture. Dev Brain Res 12:159–165
Sherrington CS (1906) The integrative action of the nervous system. Constable London
Taxt T (1983a) Motor unit numbers, motor unit sizes and innervation of single muscle fibres in hyperinnervated adult mouse soleus muscles. Acta Physiol Scand 117:571–580
Taxt T (1983b) Local and systemic effects of tetrodotoxin on the formation and elimination of synapses in reinnervated adult rat muscle. J Physiol (Lond) 340:175–194
Thompson W (1978) Reinnervation of partially denervated rat soleus muscles. Acta Physiol Scand 103:81–91
Thompson W (1983) Synapse elimination in neonatal muscle is sensitive to pattern of muscle use. Nature 302:614–616
Thompson W, Jansen JKS (1977) The extent of sprouting of remaining motor units in partly denervated immature and adult rat soleus muscle. Neuroscience 2:523–535
Thompson W, Kuffler DP, Jansen JKS (1979) The effect of prolonged reversible block of nerve impulses on the elimination of polyneuronal innervation of new-born rat skeletal muscle fibres. Neuroscience 4:271–281
Tsukuhara N (1981) Synaptic plasticity in the mammalian central nervous system. Annu Rev Neurosci 4:351–379

Electrical Activity in Injured Peripheral Nerves*

T. GORDON and L. DAVIS[1]

Nerve fiber damage elicits a response in the parent neuron and its supporting cells which is often also accompanied by an infiltration of blood-borne cells. The extent and character of this response is related to the nature, site, and severity of the injury which may vary enormously, even under controlled experimental conditions. This paper is concerned primarily with the reaction of the parent neuron to damage and the relation of functional changes in the neuron to repair and regeneration of the lost axon and to alterations in the level of neural activity.

Cellular Reaction to Nerve Fiber Injury

Classification of Injuries

Peripheral nerve injuries have been classified into three fundamental types on the basis of the extent of interruption of the nerve fiber at the lesion site: 1) compression injuries which disrupt the myelin sheath without an interruption of axon continuity and result in variable conduction failures; 2) crush injuries in which the axon is severed, but the endoneurial, epineurial, and perineurial sheaths are left intact with preservation of the normal architecture of the nerve; 3) cut injuries in which the peripheral nerve is severed such that the axon and its supporting connective tissue structures are disrupted and thereby destroy the normal architecture.

Response of Schwann Cells and Other Phagocytic Cells

The initial stages in the cellular response are occupied by overlapping degenerative and regenerative processes. Schwann cells and infiltrating phagocytic cells are involved in the compression injuries to remove damaged tissue. The proliferating Schwann cells later remyelinate the axons, and the conduction of nerve impulses resumes normally unless Schwann cell remyelination is defective (Ochoa et al. 1972). The Schwann cells also play a key role in the reaction in the crush and cut injuries where the axon continuity is disrupted. They are largely responsible for the phagocytosis of the axon debris which results from Wallerian degeneration and guidance of regenerating axons at the later stages of the reaction (Nathaniel and Pease 1963a, b).

* This work was supported by the Medical Research Council of Canada

1 Departments of Pharmacology and Orthopedic Surgery, University of Alberta, Edmonton, Alberta, T6G 2H7, Canada

Electrical Stimulation and Neuromuscular Disorders
Ed. by W. A. Nix and G. Vrbová

Response of Perineuronal Glial Cells

The perineuronal glial cells which surround the neuronal cell bodies also proliferate in response to neuronal damage. Their proliferation coincides with the retrograde changes in the neuron and may have an important nutrient function for regeneration by providing new routes of transport between neurons and blood vessels (Sjostrand 1966). Their proliferation may be triggered by changes in the dendrites of the injured neuron (Watson 1972) and, in turn, may significantly decrease neuronal activity by physically displacing synaptic boutons (Sumner 1975; Mathews and Nelson 1975).

Response of the Axotomized Neuron: Retrograde Nerve Reaction

Neurons undergo a spectrum of biochemical, structural, and functional changes following axotomy or severance of the axon. These are often collectively referred to as the chromatolytic response. Chromatolysis, strictly speaking, describes the morphological alterations that affect the nucleus, nucleolus, and Nissl granules in many, but not all, injured neurons. Detailed descriptions of the chromatolytic response were made by Lieberman (1971) and more recently by Barron (1983). The structural alterations together with other changes occurring in the parent neuron have also been referred to as the retrograde nerve reaction (Sunderland 1978), which implies that the nerve may obtain a trigger signal from the injury site. The nature of such a signal and the mechanisms of the retrograde reaction are still poorly understood, although the reaction has been viewed by several workers as an anabolic response of the neuron, appropriate for repair of the cellular damage and regeneration of the lost axon (Grafstein and McQuarrie 1978; Sunderland 1978; Gordon 1983).

There are a number of regressive changes which occur in the axotomized neurons, the denervated microenvironment of the distal nerve stump, and the denervated end-organs which result in substantial shrinkage or atrophy of the cells. The extent of these atrophic changes is controversial, and it is still unclear whether atrophic changes are progressive with time and culminate in the eventual degeneration of the cells, as has been frequently assumed (Tower 1939; Gutmann 1971). How these changes might be reconciled with cellular repair, restoration of the lost axon, and recovery of peripheral end-organs is also an open question. The answer is of obvious importance for the management of peripheral nerve injuries where recovery of function requires full recovery of the nerve, the supporting cells, and the reinnervated tissues from the denervation effects. Since nerves and muscles withdraw from the cell cycle after differentiation and do not undergo cellular division and replacement during adult life, recovery in the nerve, in particular, depends on the regenerative response, which in turn must depend on the survival of the cells.

Disuse Atrophy in Axotomized Neurons?

A loss of muscle activity in denervated muscle is probably a major factor responsible for denervation hypersensitivity and may account for some of the muscle atrophy

(Vrbová et al. 1978). We carried out experiments to determine in the first instance whether axotomized neurons continue to generate electrical activity and secondly, whether changes in activity may be a factor contributing to axonal atrophy, by analogy with disuse and denervation atrophy in skeletal muscle.

Neuronal Activity Following Axotomy

Locomotion

We implanted extracellular electrodes contained in cuffs around the sciatic nerve and one or more of its branches as well as EMG probes on extensor and flexor muscles in hindlimbs of cats as described in detail previously (Davis et al. 1978; Gordon and Stein 1982). The cables were led via a percutaneous plug to amplifiers for recording of nerve and muscle signals in the freely moving cat. Reciprocal activation of flexor and extensor nerves and muscles was recorded during locomotion of the normal cat on a treadmill. The sensory and motor components of the neural signals were extracted by a method of cross-correlation of the signals recorded on the nerve at two points, as described by Gordon et al. (1980) and Stein et al. (1981). Figure 1 shows

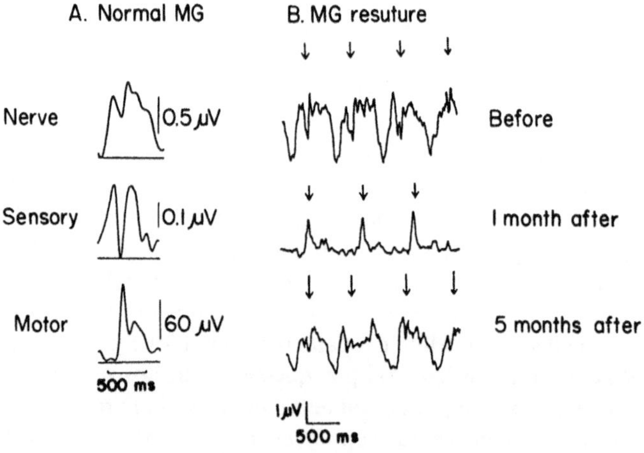

Fig. 1A, B. Pattern of activity (after rectification and filtering) of the nerve which supplies the medial gastrocnemius *(MG)* muscle of the extensor group in the cat hindlimb, during locomotion on a treadmill. **B** The activity was recorded by extracellular recording electrodes contained in cuffs around the MG nerve prior to sectioning and surgically uniting the proximal and distal stumps, 1 month and 5 months after the operation. Timing of the bursts of activity were reproducible from step to step with activity beginning before foot fall (↓) and maintained during the extensor phase of locomotion. **A** The average burst pattern for a number of step cycles beginning with the flexor phase was subdivided into sensory and motor components. Sensory activity was extracted by analog multiplication of neural signals on the MG and sciatic nerves with the appropriate delay obtained from cross-correlation. Motor signals were similarly obtained and resembled closely the EMG pattern from the MG muscle. Note that in **B** the extensor burst pattern closely resembles the motor component and that the more complex pattern of motor and sensory activity returns 5 months after MG resuture after sensory and motor reinnervation has taken place (from Gordon et al. 1980; Stein et al. 1981)

the rhythmical activity of an extensor nerve which supplies the medial gastrocnemius (MG) muscle. When neural activity and its sensory component during the extensor phase of stepping is averaged together with EMG activity for several steps, it is clear that much of the characteristic neural discharge is sensory. Within weeks of axotomy this sensory component is completely lost in the nerves proximal to the injury site. In contrast, the motor nerves continue to generate a pattern of activity characteristic of the motor discharge of the normal nerve. The decline in the neural signal is in part accounted for by sensory loss. In addition, measurement of the motor component from cross-correlogram functions showed that motor activity also declined during the first month after axotomy (Gordon et al 1980). Nevertheless, motor activity was never completely lost, and axotomized motor axons continued to generate appropriate patterns of activity of lower but stable amplitude during locomotion. This was so even one year after cutting and ligating the nerve to prevent regeneration of the axons and reinnervation of the target organs.

Although the general form of the flexor and extensor activity is qualitatively normal, changes in synaptic input and neuronal properties following axotomy lead to a significant change in the firing patterns of the neurons and a reduction in the amplitude of the neural signals.

Dysjunction of Synapses and Pattern of Discharge

In order to study the effect of axotomy on the excitable properties of neurons, we have used the bullfrog sympathetic ganglionic neurons as a model because of their viability *in vitro* for detailed intracellular recordings and in order to extend these studies to the investigation of the role of nerve growth factor in maintenance of normal neuronal properties and axonal dimensions. We found that stimulation of preganglionic neurons normally evoked a postsynaptic response in the postganglionic neurons but sometimes failed to evoke a response in axotomized neurons. Findings of synaptic depression in axotomized neurons in mammalian sympathetic ganglia (Purves 1975) and mammalian and amphibian motoneurons (Mendell et al. 1976; Shapovalov and Grantyn 1968) are consistent with morphological data of displacement of synaptic boutons from the cell bodies and dendrites (e.g. Summer 1975; Mathews and Nelson 1975). The time of synaptic dysfunction in motoneurons readily accounts for the rapid decline in efferent signals after axotomy (Gordon et al. 1980).

A rapid and dramatic change in the duration of the action potential within 2 weeks of cutting the postganglionic nerves, 2–8 mm from the ganglia, significantly alters the discharge of the neuron to excitatory input (Fig. 2). Normally, activation of Ca^{2+}-sensitive potassium conductance by Ca^{2+} entering the cell during the action potential hyperpolarizes the neuron for up to 200 ms. This afterhyperpolarization (AHP) limits the firing frequency and prevents repetitive firing during maintained excitation or a depolarizing current (accommodation) (Kernell 1983). A 40% reduction in AHP amplitude and a 70% reduction in the AHP duration in the axotomized neuron was associated with less accommodation in the neurons which discharged more rapidly and repetitively in response to maintained excitatory input (Smith et al. 1985). Repetitive firing in response to synaptic input might compensate for loss of some synaptic terminals and thereby maintain the activity of the neurons.

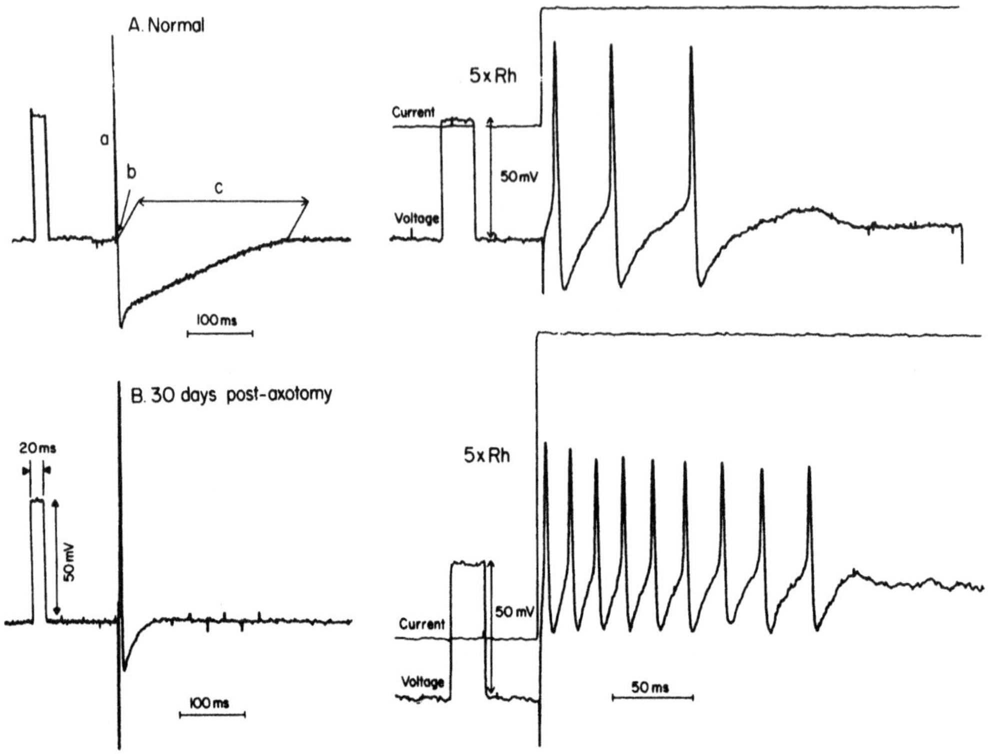

Fig. 2A, B. Antidromic action potentials and action potentials evoked by current injection were recorded with standard intracellular recording techniques in the postganglionic neurons of the IXth and Xth sympathetic ganglia in **A** normal bullfrogs *(Rana catesbeiana)* and **B** 30 days after section of the postganglionic nerves 2–8 mm from the ganglion. Stimulation of cut end of the postganglionic fibres with suction electrodes elicited an antidromic spike *(a)* which was followed by a prominent afterhyperpolarization (AHP) which decayed to resting potential. AHP duration, measured between *b* and *c* was dramatically reduced after axotomy, and axotomized neurones fired spikes more frequently and more rapidly in response to a 5x rheobase current step

Neuronal Atrophy

The correlation of nerve and muscle atrophy with the decline in levels of neural activity might suggest disuse as a causative factor responsible, at least in part, for atrophy of nerve and muscle cells. The characteristic time course and extent of atrophy in axotomized neurons and denervated muscle fibers show striking similarities: size of nerve and muscle fibers declines most rapidly immediately following the lesion. The atrophy follows an exponential time course to reach a final stable level of 20% and 28% of normal in nerve and muscle fibers, with time constants (τ) of 29 and 46 days, respectively (Fig. 3). There was no evidence for a progressive deterioration culminating in degeneration, and cell numbers showed no significant change from normal.

The most rapid decline of neural potential in cut cat nerves coincides with the most rapid decline in neural activity during locomotion (Gordon et al. 1980). Is the

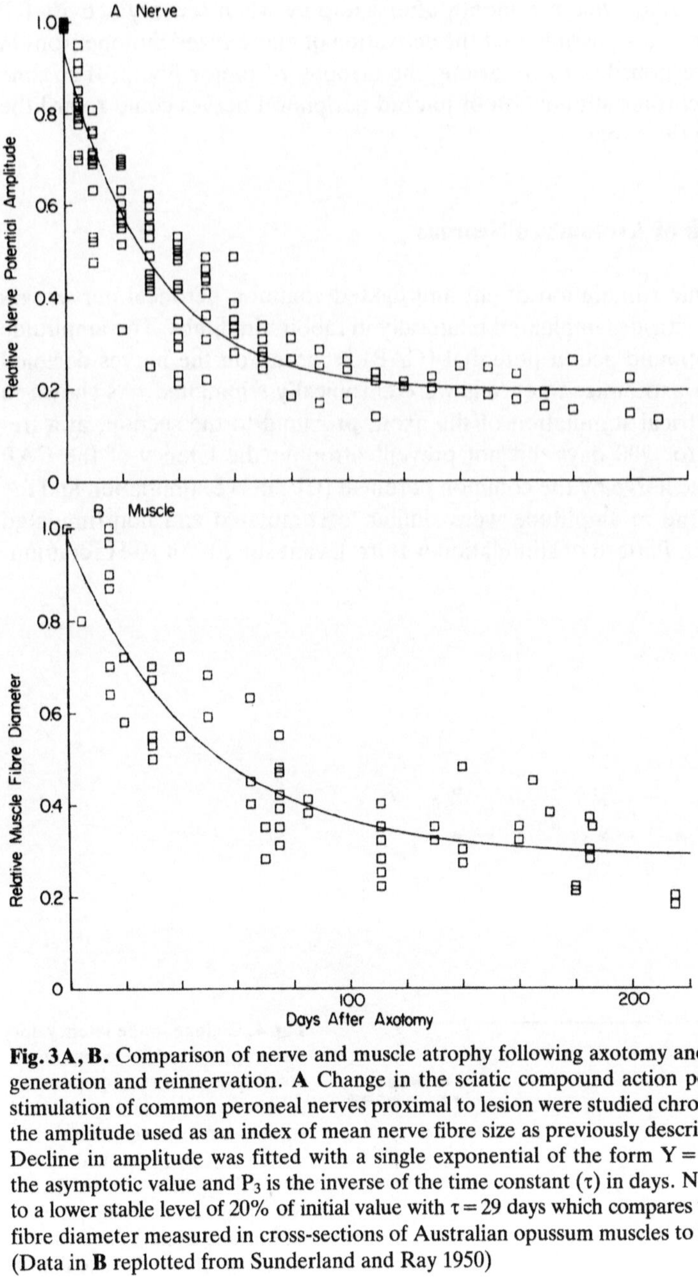

Fig. 3A, B. Comparison of nerve and muscle atrophy following axotomy and ligation to prevent regeneration and reinnervation. **A** Change in the sciatic compound action potentials in response to stimulation of common peroneal nerves proximal to lesion were studied chronically in 10 rabbits and the amplitude used as an index of mean nerve fibre size as previously described (Davis et al. 1978). Decline in amplitude was fitted with a single exponential of the form $Y = P_1 + P_2e^{P_3x}$ where P_1 is the asymptotic value and P_3 is the inverse of the time constant (τ) in days. Nerve amplitude declines to a lower stable level of 20% of initial value with $\tau = 29$ days which compares with **B** decline in muscle fibre diameter measured in cross-sections of Australian opussum muscles to 28% with a $\tau = 47$ days. (Data in **B** replotted from Sunderland and Ray 1950)

atrophy and relative disuse causally related? Sensory fibers become quiescent within a month and do not discharge again unless they reinnervate target organs. These fibers undergo significantly greater atrophy than motor fibers (Hoffer et al. 1979) which would be consistent with disuse atrophy of sensory fibres and lesser atrophy in the more active motor fibers. Interestingly, the relatively greater atrophy of the sensory axons only became evident a month after axotomy when sensory activity fell below motor activity. It is possible that the activation of axotomized motoneurons in the spinal cord is responsible for retarding the atrophy of motor fibers. If so, one might predict that chronic stimulation of injured peripheral nerves could retard the atrophic changes in the axons.

Chronic Stimulation of Axotomized Neurons

The effect of chronic stimulation of cut and ligated common peroneal nerves was studied with cuff electrodes implanted bilaterally in rabbit hindlimbs. The amplitude of the evoked compound action potential (CAP) recorded on the nerves declined whether or not the axotomized neurons were chronically stimulated. As shown in Fig. 4, chronic electrical stimulation of the axon, proximal to the section, at a frequency of 8 h/day for 200 days did not prevent atrophy: the latency of the CAP evoked on the sciatic nerve by the common peroneal (CP) nerve stimulation and the accompanying decline in amplitude were similar in stimulated and nonstimulated axotomized neurons. Pattern of stimulation was irrelevant since both 10-Hz continu-

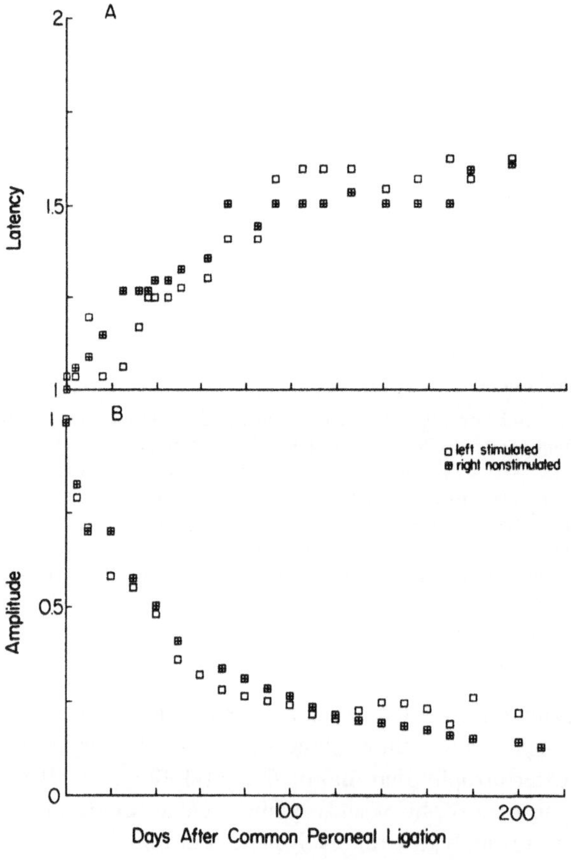

Fig. 4. Change in the latency and the amplitude of the compound action potential recorded on sciatic nerves evoked by maximal stimulation of the common peroneal (CP) nerve, with time after CP ligation. Control data was obtained bilaterally prior to cutting and ligating the CP nerve bilaterally 10 mm distal to the CP cuff electrode, and commencing chronic electrical stimulation of the left CP nerve (□) daily for 8 h with pulses at 10 Hz. The right ligated CP nerve (⊞) served as the control

ous and 100-Hz intermittent stimulation were ineffective in reversing nerve fiber atrophy.

These experiments show that axonal atrophy and decline in neural activity are sequelae to axotomy but unlikely to be casually related. Consequently, replacement of neural activity with electrical stimulation will not prevent the atrophy.

Neuronal Atrophy and Its Relation to Regeneration

Loss of Axoplasm

A simple explanation for axonal atrophy was offered by Gutmann and Sanders in 1943. A decline in nerve fiber diameter proximal to the injury might be the consequence of an outflow of axoplasm into the elongating axons which have sprouted from the cut axons. If this were the case, atrophy of nerve fibers would occur only when axons are being regenerated. However, we found that axonal atrophy was similar and followed the same time course in axotomized neurons which were ligated to prevent regeneration and elongation as in neurons which were encouraged to regenerate after nerve repair (Davis et al. 1978). Axoplasm is therefore not simply lost to sprouting axons from the parent axon.

Axonal Transport

There is now considerable evidence for a synthesis in the cell body of axotomized neurons of material for cell growth and transport to the growing axons (reviewed by Grafstein and McQuarrie 1978). Cytoskeletal proteins which provide the motility of the growth cone are transported in relatively higher quantitites in regenerating axons than normal (Hoffman and Lasek 1980). The relative decline in neurofilament transport may provide a reasonable explanation for the axonal atrophy, because the axon diameter has been correlated with the content of neurofilaments.

Reformation of Neuronal Connections

An attractive hypothesis outlined by Lasek and Black (1977) suggests that the axonal process of a mature neuron is in a constant state of growth as a consequence of a continual transport of cytoskeletal proteins from the cell body. This growth is halted at its terminal contracts by a breakdown of the proteins in the nerve terminals. When the neuron is sectioned, regeneration of the lost axon reflects unimpeded progression of the cytoskeleton and synthesis of axolemma from membrane transported by fast axonal transport. Recognition of the target again halts growth and the greater transport of neurofilaments allows for a maturation of the axons with an increase in their diameter. The same motor fiber population of cat hindlimb nerves was sampled before and after nerve section and surgical repair as described elsewhere (Gordon

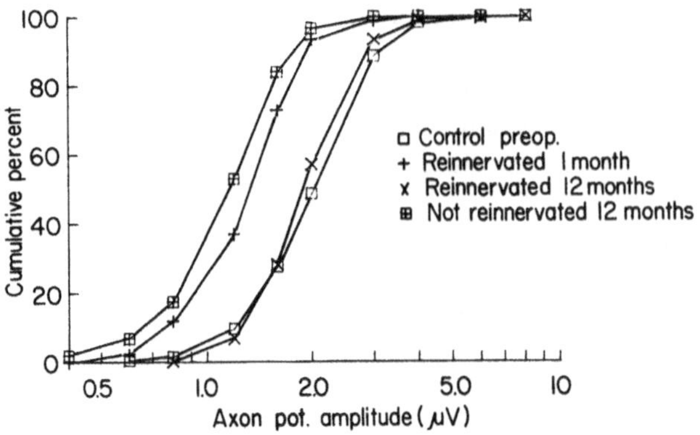

Fig. 5. Cumulative probability distribution of axon potential amplitudes recorded from the same axonal population, before (□), 2 to 3 months (+) and 1 year after nerve section and suture (× and ⊞) (from Gordon and Stein 1982). Axon potential amplitudes recorded proximal to the injury site were smaller than normal when regenerating axons first made functional nerve-muscle connections (+) but recovered fully (×). Axons which did not remake nerve-muscle contacts (⊞) remained significantly smaller than normal. Note that all motor axons were similarly affected by denervation and reinnervation. (From Gordon 1983)

and Stein 1982) to determine atrophy in single axons and the effect of reinnervation on nerve fibers. We found that the nerve fibers atrophied following axotomy but could fully recover their former size if regenerating axons made functional nerve-muscle contacts as shown by the overlap of cumulative frequency histogram of reinnervated motor fibers with that of the same fibers before peripheral nerve section (Fig. 5). The time course of recovery was correlated directly with recovery of the reinnervated muscle units (Gordon and Stein 1982). These findings argued strongly for a retrograde control of the nerve fiber diameter from the end organ and is consistent with the idea that elaboration of a nerve terminal halts growth.

Role of Calcium

The influx of calcium into the terminal activates a protease which may be responsible for the breakdown of cytoskeletal proteins (Schlaepfer and Hasler 1979). Calcium ions are ubiquitous in cellular control mechanisms. They are probably involved in normal axonal transport in neurons (Ochs 1982) and are implicated in cellular movement in a wide variety of cells. They also appear to have a pivotal role in the movement of growth cones of growing nerves (Suarez-Gsla et al. 1984). Our recent experiments on bullfrog sympathetic neurons indicate that axotomy promotes a loss of calcium-sensitive slow potassium conductance in the cell body without affecting the calcium channels (Smith et al. 1985; Kelly et al. 1985). This is seen as a decrease in AHP duration and amplitude, a widening of the antidromic spikes, and a decreased accommodation to depolarizing current (cf. Fig. 2). Since there are still calcium channels in the membranes of axotomized neurons, the loss of Ca-sensitive potassium conductance may be explained by intracellular sequestration of the calcium or alterations in the potassium channels themselves.

These changes occur rapidly after an initial delay of up to 6 days following axotomy of the ganglionic cells. Within 2 weeks, the AHP duration was significantly shorter and remained stable thereafter, unless peripheral contacts were reformed (Smith et al. 1985). The delay may correspond to the latent period which proceeds outgrowth of regenerating sprouts from cut nerves and the rapid fall in AHP duration may coincide with transport of altered proportions of cytoskeletal proteins for extension of the growth cones.

Conclusion

It is tempting to speculate firstly that altered calcium handling of the axotomized cell may be involved in the regenerative response of the axotomized cell and that secondly, the atrophy which progresses rapidly in the first month after nerve injury reflects a dedifferentiation of the neuron to a growing state which may be readily reversed by reformation of peripheral contacts.

Acknowledgements. The research was carried out in collaboration with Drs. Hoffer, Jhamandas, Kelly, Orosco, Smith and Stein, Ms. Susan Buller, Mr. G. Goldsand and J. Shapiro.

References

Barron KD (1983) Comparative observations on the cytologic reactions of central and peripheral nerve cells to axotomy. In: Kao CC, Bunge RP, Reier RJ (eds) Spinal cord reconstruction. Raven, New York, pp 7–40

Davis LA, Gordon T, Hoffer JA, Jhamandas J, Stein RB (1978) Compound action potentials recorded from mammalian peripheral nerves following ligation or resuturing. J Physiol 285: 543–559

Gordon T (1983) Dependence of peripheral nerves on their target organs. In: Burnstock G, Vrbová G, O'Brien R (eds) Somatic and autonomic nerve-muscle interactions. Elsevier, Amsterdam, pp 289–235

Gordon T, Stein RB (1982) Time course and extent of recovery in reinnervated motor units of cat triceps surae muscles. J Physiol 323: 307–323

Gordon T, Hoffer JA, Jhamandas J, Stein RB (1980) Long-term effects of axotomy on neural activity during cat locomotion. J Physiol 303: 243–263

Grafstein B, McQuarrie IG (1978) The role of the nerve cell body in axon regeneration. In: Cotman C (ed) Neuronal plasticity. Raven, New York, pp 155–195

Gutmann E (1971) Histology of degeneration and regeneration. In: Licht (ed) Electrodiagnosis and electromyography, 3rd edn. Published by the Editor, New Haven, pp 113–133

Gutmann E, Sanders FK (1943) Recovery of fibre numbers and diameters in the regeneration of peripheral nerves. J Physiol 101: 489–518

Hoffer JA, Stein RB, Gordon T (1979) Differential atrophy of sensory and motor fibers following section of cat peripheral nerves. Brain Res 178: 347–361

Hoffman PL, Lasek RJ (1980) Axonal transport of the cytoskeleton in regenerating motor neurons: constancy and change. Brain Res 202: 317–333

Kelly MEM, Shapiro J, Smith PA, Gordon T (1985) Axotomy attenuates Ca^{2+}-sensitive potassium conductance (g_K) in amphibian sympathetic neurons. In: XX Canadian congress of neurol sci. (to be published)

Kernell D (1983) Functional properties of spinal motoneurons and gradation of muscle force. In: Desmedt JE (ed) Motor control mechanisms in health and disease. Raven, New York, pp 213–226

Lasek RJ, Black MM (1977) How do axons stop growing? Some clues from the metabolism of the proteins in the slow component of axonal transport. In: Roberts et al. (eds) Mechanisms, regulation and special functions of protein synthesis in the brain. Elsevier/North-Holland Biomedical Press, Amsterdam, pp 161–169

Lieberman AR (1971) The axon reaction: a review of the principal features of perikaryal response to axon injury. Int Rev Neurobiol 14:49–124

Mathews MR, Nelson VH (1975) Detachment of structurally intact nerve endings from chromatolytic neurones of rat superior cervical ganglion during the depression of synaptic transmission induced by post-ganglionic axotomy. J Physiol 245:91–135

Mendell LM, Munson JB, Scott JG (1976) Alterations of synapses on axotomized motoneurons. J Physiol 255:67–79

Nathaniel EJH, Pease DC (1963a) Degenerative changes in rat dorsal roots during Wallerian degeneration. J Ultrastruct Res 9:511–532

Nathaniel EJH, Pease DC (1963b) Regenerative changes in rat dorsal roots following Wallerian degeneration. J Ultrastruct Res 9:533–549

Ochoa J, Fowler TJ, Gilliatt RW (1972) Anatomical changes in peripheral nerves compressed by a pneumatic tourniquet. J Anat 113:433–455

Ochs S (1982) Axoplasmic transport and its relation to nerve function. Wiley, New York

Purves D (1975) Functional and structural changes of mammalian sympathetic neurones following interruption of their axons. J Physiol 252:429–463

Schlaepfer WW, Hasler MB (1979) Characterization of the calcium-induced disruption of neurofilaments in rat peripheral nerve. Brain Res 168:299–309

Shapovalov AI, Grantyn AA (1968) Suprasegmental synaptic influences on chromatolyzed motor neurones. Biophysics 13:308–319

Sjostrand J (1966) Studies on glial cells in the hypoglossal nucleus of the rabbit during nerve regeneration. Act Physiol Scand 67 [Suppl]:270

Smith PA, Shapiro J, Kelly MEM, Gordon T (1985) Effect of axotomy on Ca^{2+}-sensitive potassium conductance (g_K) in sympathetic ganglia. Can Fed Biol Soc 28:92

Stein RB, Gordon T, Oguztoreli MN, Lee RG (1981) Classifying sensory patterns and their effects on locomotion and tremor. Can J Physiol Pharmacol 59:645–655

Suarez-Gsla BA, Pelto DJ, Thompson JM, Rapoport SI (1984) Blockers of calcium permeability inhibit neurite extension and formation of neuromuscular synapses in cell culture. Dev Brain Res 14:263–270

Sumner BEH (1975) A quantitative analysis of the response of presynaptic boutons to post synaptic motor axotomy. Exp Neurol 46:605–615

Sunderland S (1978) Nerves and nerve injuries. Livingstone, Edinburgh

Sunderland S, Ray LJ (1950) Denervation changes in mammalian striated muscle. J Neurol Neurosurg Psychiatry 13:159–177

Tower SS (1939) The reaction of muscle to denervation. Physiol Rev 19:1–48

Vrbová G, Gordon T, Jones R (1978) Nerve-muscle interaction. Chapman and Hall, London

Watson WE (1972) Some quantitative observations upon the responses of neuraglial cells which follow axotomy of adjacent neurons. J Physiol 225:415–435

Assessment of the Regenerative Capacity of Peripheral Nervous System: Enhancement of Sprouting Capacity by Exogenous Gangliosides

M. Vitadello[1,2], C. Triban[1], P. Marini[1], R. Zanoni[1], M. Fabris[1], and A. Gorio[1]

Following a nerve crush, the distal segment degenerates while a retrograde reaction is induced in the neuronal cell body (chromatolysis) and accompanied by modification of protein metabolism. Such a response is possibly related to the regenerative process: in fact, elongation of regenerating axons occurs at the tip of neuronal sprouts by the addition of new material brought by axonal transport. Previous studies have demonstrated a decrease of the anterograde fast axonal flow of enzymes, associated with synaptic transmission, within 1–2 days of axotomy (Heiwall et al. 1979; O'Brien 1978). Other axonal constituents carried with fast transport are not necessarily decreased, since the total amount of fast transported protein may increase after axotomy (see Grafstein and Forman 1980; for a review). Concerning slow transport, which conveys most of cytoskeletal constituents of axons, changes in both rate and composition of the related transported molecules have been described (Hoffmann and Lasek 1980; Skene and Willard 1981). The regenerative process of a nerve implies the reconstitution of morphological and structural properties of injured axons accompanied by the restoration of functional activity. Keeping these problems in mind, the time course of the regeneration of crushed rat sciatic nerve has been studied. In particular, the elongation of injured axons was followed by the immunohistochemical tracing of the 145 K neurofilament polypeptide (Vitadello et al. 1986) at the level of the crush site and of the homolateral extensor digitorum longus (EDL) muscle. The functional recovery of the regenerating nerve was monitored by the measurement of the anterograde axonal flow of the transmission-related enzyme acetylcholinesterase (AChE, E.C. 3.1.1.7.) in the proximal nerve stump. Finally, the reappearance of miniature end plate potentials (mepp) in the denervated EDL muscle fibers was monitored electrophysiologically at different times after sciatic nerve crush. Experiments were carried out on 180–200 g albino Sprague Dawley rats. The sciatic nerve was crushed just before the gluteal branching. As a measure of AChE axonal transport we used the accumulation of this enzyme over a 24-h period at a test section of the parent nerve (see Fig. 1 for experimental details). AChE flow was already decreased 24 h after crush, reached its minimal level on day 4, then recovered gradually to control level between 30 and 60 days (Fig. 1).

Indirect immunofluorescence staining of regenerating axons was performed by means of iC8, a monoclonal antibody specific for the 145K subunit of the neurofilament triplet in rat sciatic nerve (Vitadello et al. 1986). Results showed a population of axons growing through the crush site as early as 3 days after the lesion (Fig. 2). Immunoblotting experiments on crushed nerves showed that immunoreactivity dis-

1 FIDIA Research Laboratories, Via Ponte della Fabbrica 3/a, 35031 Abano Terme, Italy
2 Present address: Istituto Fisiologia Centri Nervosi – CNR –, Via Mario Bianco 9, 20131 Milano, Italy

Electrical Stimulation and Neuromuscular Disorders
Ed. by W. A. Nix and G. Vrbová

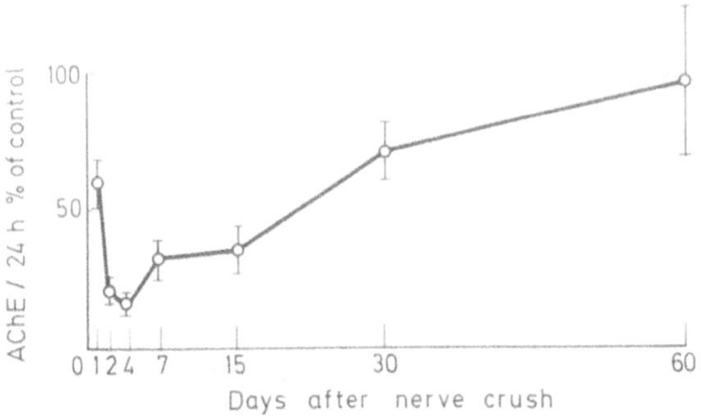

Fig. 1. Evaluation of the anterograde accumulation rate of AChE in crushed rat sciatic nerve. At several times after crush the accumulation rate of AChE was measured in the proximal stump by the nerve section method (Couraud and Di Giamberardino 1980). The nerve was sectioned 3–5 mm proximal to the nerve crush and the enzyme was allowed to accumulate. AChE activity was measured 24 h later in the 2-mm nerve segment proximal to the section. Each segment was homogenized in 200 µl of extraction buffer (1 *M* NaCl, 0.01 *M* phosphate buffer pH 7.0, 0.05 m*M* EGTA, 1% Triton X100, 1 mg/ml bacitracin, 2 m*M* benzamidine). After centrifugation (20000 × g, 20 min), AChE activity was assayed on the supernatant using 0.75 m*M* acetylthiocholine as substrate and 0.1 m*M* iso-OMPA as pseudocholinesterase inhibitor. The anterograde accumulation rate of AChE was defined as the quantity of enzyme, beyond that normally present in the nerve, accumulated over a 24-h period at the 2-mm nerve segment proximal to the section. Control accumulation rates were measured in sciatic nerves of uncrushed rats of the same age. Each *point* represents the mean of at least three determinations

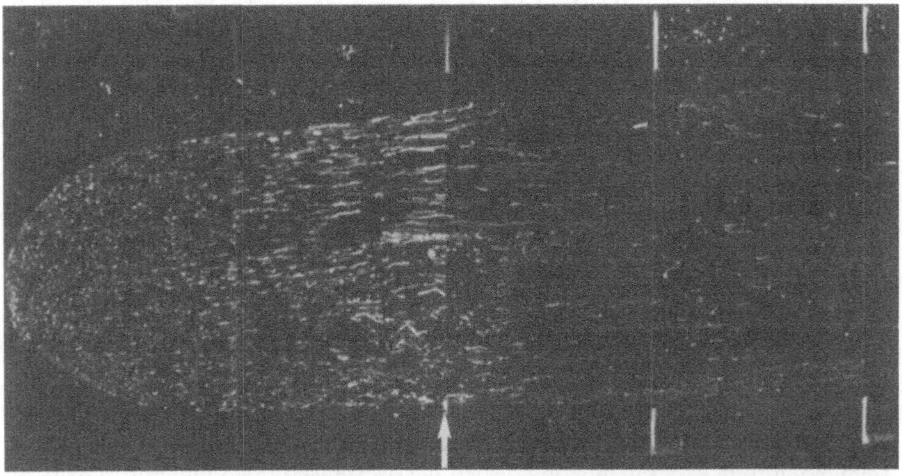

Fig. 2. Indirect immunofluorescence staining with antineurofilament mAb iC8 of rat sciatic nerve 3 days after crush. The *arrow* indicates the crush site: a normal pattern of reactivity was seen proximal to the lesion *(left)*. Distally, only granular debris with NF immunoreactivity were observed. In addition, tiny processes growing through the crush were labelled; they were interpreted as regenerating axons

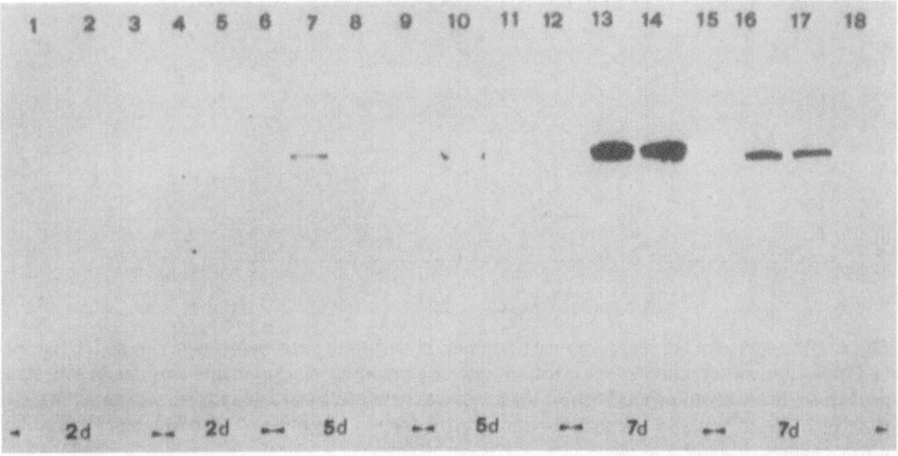

Fig. 3. Immunoblots of rat sciatic nerve homogenates at different distances (0–3 mm: lanes 1–4–7–10–13–16; 3–6 mm: lanes 2–5–8–11–14–17; 10–13 mm: lanes 3–6–9–12–15–18) from the crush site, 2–5–7 days after lesion. Nerve segments were homogenated in sample buffer (3% SDS 65 m*M* Tris-HCl, 5 m*M* EGTA, 5% 2-mercaptoethanol pH 6.8) and polypeptides were separated on 7.5%–15% acrilamide gradient by SDS-PAGE (Laemmli 1970). Proteins were transferred to nitrocellulose paper, which was incubated with iC8 and then with ^{125}I rabbit anti-mouse IgG. Dried blots were set for autoradiography with Kodak-X-O-MAT films. Two days after crush the 145K NF subunit disappeared distally to the crush site, by day 5 immunoreactivity was detected in 0–3 mm nerve segments and by day 7 also in the 3–6 mm nerve segments distal to the crush

appeared distally to the crush site 2 days after the lesion; 5 days after the crush immunoreactivity was detected in the first 3 mm nerve segment distal to the crush site and by day 7 also in the 2nd 3-mm nerve segment (Fig. 3). Immunohistochemical examination of the denervated EDL muscle revealed no labeled axon 4 days after sciatic nerve lesion; tiny fibers innervating neuromuscular junctions were decorated by anti-neurofilament antibody by day 15 after nerve injury, indicating that regenerating motor axons were reaching their target. At this time, electrophysiological recording of EDL muscle fibers revealed the reappearance of miniature end plate potentials at a rate of about 1 per minute. The frequency gradually increased with time and reached control values 40 days after crush (Fig. 4).

Our results showed that restoration of synaptic transmission occurred when regenerating axons, labeled with anti-neurofilament antibody, reached the neuromuscular junction in the EDL muscle. This fact may indicate that neurofilament polypeptides travel down growing axons at a velocity very close to that of regenerating axons. The study of slow transport velocity in regenerating sciatic nerve motor axons showed no change in parent axons, although changes in the amount of material in the two subcomponents of slow transport were found (Hoffmann and Lasek 1980). However, the precise role of slow transport in axonal elongation cannot be elucidated until more is known about slow transport mechanism and how transported material is deployed in regenerating axons. For example, the fact that regenerating axons are much thinner beyond the lesion level might suggest that axonal outgrowth may depend, to some extent, on the diversion and reutilization of materials that normally

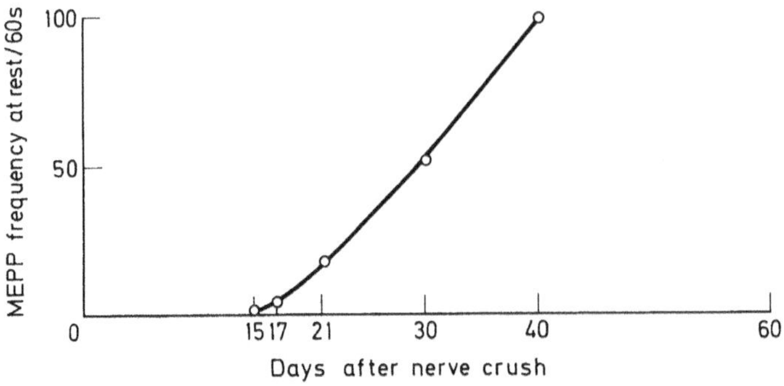

Fig. 4. Time course of the reappearance of miniature end plate potentials (mepp) in the EDL muscle at various times after sciatic nerve crush. Membrane potential measurements were made with standard intracellular recording techniques. No mepp was detected before day 15 after lesion, then mepps were recorded at very low frequency in newly reinnervated end plates. Mepp frequency returned to normal values in about 4 weeks

Table 1. Extent of collateral reinnervation of soleus muscle 30 days after resection of L_5

MU	R	RT
1	15.0 ± 3.1 (5)	21.0 ± 1.0 (8)
2	27.7 ± 3.0 (6)	42.0 ± 2.0 (4)
5	63.0 ± 3.5 (5)	86.0 ± 3.9 (5)
8	89.6 ± 3.2 (4)	97.0 ± 1.9 (6)

MU, number of motor units remaining after L_5 section; R, tension developed by reinnervated muscles; RT, tension developed by reinnervated muscles from animals treated with gangliosides

maintain the caliber of axons proximal to the injury site (Hoffmann et al. 1984). It is interesting to note that the anterograde axonal transport of AChE was still at its minimal level when a population of crushed axons began to grow across the lesion site. On the other hand, AChE orthograde axonal flow began to recover before regenerating axons reached the neuromuscular junction, as indicated by immunohistochemical and electrophysiological methods, suggesting that the recovery of AChE transport must precede reinnervation. Furthermore, this parameter could be used as a marker for a positive recovery, in agreement no restoration of AChE anterograde axonal flow was detected in cut nerves (Di Giamberardino et al. 1981). Thus, the determination of AChE axonal flow might prove quite important in testing the effects of drugs or surgical procedures of nerve repair on peripheral nerve regeneration.

In another set of experiments we assessed the effects of the administration of exogenous gangliosides on motoneuron sprouting capacity. Rat soleus muscle was partially denervated by resecting L5 mixed-nerve. The proximal stump of the resected nerve was ligated and the distal stump was sutured intraperitoneally. At various times after surgery animals were examined and the extent of recovery was estimated by comparing maximal isometric tension of the denervated soleus muscle with that of the undenervated controlateral one. The number of motor units still remaining after L5 resection was determined by stimulating the nerve with increasing electric currents. The gradual recruitment of motoneurons resulted in a gradual stepwise increase of muscle tension up to a plateau; the simple counting of tension steps gave a direct estimate of motor units innervating the soleus muscle. Results showed that motor units can expand their peripheral field after partial denervation of the muscle (Table 1); daily intraperitoneal injections with 5 mg/g gangliosides (GM_1; 21%, GD_{Ia} 39.7%; GD_{1B} 16% and GT 19%) enhanced the sprouting capacity and consequently the reinnervating capacity of surviving motor axons. For instance, if, after L5 resection, only one functional motor unit remains in soleus muscle, the tension developed by the muscle from untreated and treated rats is, respectively, 15% and 21% of the tension developed by contralateral undenervated muscle. This result is in accordance with previous reports indicating that gangliosides are accumulated in the sciatic nerve and stimulated neuronal sprouting after crush (Gorio et al. 1980). In addition, exogenous gangliosides stimulated NGF-induced neuritogenesis of PC_{12} cells in vitro (Ferrari et al. 1983). The precise ganglioside molecular mode of action is yet to be defined, but it seems likely that they can trigger membrane changes followed by cellular modification which make a site ready to form a new branch.

Acknowledgements. AChE axonal transport measurements were done in collaboration with Drs. L. Di Giamberardino and R. Hassig from the Département de Biologie du C.E.N. de Saclay, France.

References

Couraud JY, Di Giamberadino L (1980) Axonal transport of acetylcholinesterase in chick sciatic nerve. J Neurochem 35:1053–1066

Di Giamberardino L, Couraud JY, Hassig R, Marini P, Gorio A (1981) The use of acetylcholinesterase molecular forms to appraise post-traumatic recovery of nerve and muscle. In: Gorio A, Millesi H, Mingrino S (eds) Post-traumatic peripheral nerve regeneration. Raven, New York, pp 453–458

Ferrari G, Fabris M, Gorio A (1983) Gangliosides enhance neurite outgrowth in PC_{12} cells. Dev Brain Res 8:215–222

Gorio A, Carmignoto G, Facci L, Finesso M (1980) Motor nerve sprouting induced by ganglioside treatment. Possible implications for gangliosides of neuronal growth. Brain Res 197:236–241

Grafstein B, Forman DS (1980) Intracellular transport in neurons. Physiol Rev 60:1167–1283

Heiwall PO, Dahlstrom A, Larsson DA, Booij S (1979) The intraaxonal transport of acetylcholine and cholinergic enzymes in rat sciatic nerve during regeneration after various types of axonal trauma. J Neurobiol 10:119–136

Hoffmann PN, Lasek RJ (1980) Axonal transport of the cytoskeleton in regenerating motoneurons: constancy and changes. Brain Res 202:317–333

Hoffman PN, Griffin JW, Price DL (1984) Control of axonal caliber by neurofilament transport. J Cell Biol 99:705–714

Laemmli VK (1970) Cleavage of structural proteins during the assembly of the head of the bacteriophage T_4. Nature 227:680–685.

O'Brien RAD (1978) Axonal transport of acetylcholine, choline acetyltransferase and cholinesterase in regenerating peripheral nerve. J Physiol (Lond) 282:91–103

Skene JHP, Willard M (1981) Axonally transported proteins associated with axon growth in rabbit central and peripheral neurons system. J Cell Biol 89:96–103

Vitadello M, Triban C, Fabris M, Gorio A, Schiaffino S (1986) Heterogeneity of rat neurofilament polypeptides revealed by a monoclonal antibody. J Neurochem 46:665–670

Effects of Activity on Restorative Processes in the Autonomic Nervous System

R. Jones[1] and G. Burnstock[2]

Introduction

Numerous experimental studies indicate the importance of preganglionic nerve activity on the functional, biochemical and morphological development and maintenance of postganglionic adrenergic neurones. Spinal cord section during early postnatal development impairs the maturation of adrenergic neurones (Black et al. 1976), and in adults cold stress fails to induce an increase in tyrosine hydroxylase if preganglionic pathways are not intact and functional (Bloom et al. 1976). The role of preganglionic cholinergic neurones in the maintenance of adrenergic postganglionic cells was reviewed by Thoenen (1972), but there is little information indicating whether the influence of preganglionic neurones is mediated solely by impulse traffic or whether other factors prevail. Some authors have looked at the effects of acute electrical stimulation on this system. Zigmond and Chalazonitis (1979) for example reported that short periods of stimulation of the preganglionic cervical sympathetic trunk induced increased tyrosine hydroxylase activity in postganglionic neurones which could still be detected 72 h after stimulation. The level of this increase depended on total stimulation time. Further, Gillespie and McGrath (1974) showed that the rate of noradrenaline depletion in reserpine-treated rats was dependent on impulse traffic.

These studies indicate that the biochemical responses of adrenergic neurones are regulated by impulse traffic, but it has been suggested that the ability of cells to grow and form functional synaptic contacts is also influenced by preganglionic neural activity (Thoenen 1972; Saito et al. 1981). We wished to examine this further by studying the effect of long-term imposed electrical stimulation of preganglionic nerves on the ability of adrenergic neurones to grow and reinnervate a regenerating target organ and on the efficiency of intact target organ innervation.

Methods

Studies were carried out using the guinea pig vas deferens, which has dense adrenergic innervation of both circular and longitudinal muscle layers (Furness and Iwyama 1972).

The technique of removing a small portion of the wall of the vas deferens, mincing it under sterile conditions and returning the 'mince' to its site of origin enabled

1 Oncology Research Unit, Radiotherapy Centre, Bristol Royal Infirmary, Bristol BS2 8ED, U.K.
2 Department of Anatomy & Embryology, University College, London WC1E 6BT, U.K.

Electrical Stimulation and Neuromuscular Disorders
Ed. by W. A. Nix and G. Vrbová

us to examine the reinnervation of regenerating muscle cells in situ (Yokota et al. 1978; Burnstock et al. 1978b). Using this model the time course of reinnervation was studied on montages of electronmicrographs of the minced regenerating muscle cells. Adrenergic nerve terminals were recognised by the presence of dense cored vesicles after incubation with 5-hydroxy-dopamine (Tranzer and Thoenen 1967). The number of nerve profiles and nerve varicosities within 100 n*M* of the nearest muscle cell was counted on photomontages at different intervals after the initial operation. Results were expressed as number of nerve profiles per 100 muscle cells.

Decentralisation

Decentralisation of one vas deferens in each animal was carried out by section of the hypogastric nerve in the abdominal cavity under halothane anaesthesia using aseptic procedures.

Stimulation

Stimulation was imposed using bipolar teflon coated silver or platignum wires implanted on the hypogastric nerve with leads externalised behind the head. Continuous stimulation at 2 Hz with 0.2 ms impulses was carried out for 6–8 h daily (Burnstock et al. 1978a; Jones et al. 1983a, b).

The ipsilateral vas deferens in decentralised or stimulated preparations was either left intact, or a small portion of the vessel wall was removed, minced and returned to its site of origin as described above.

Physiology and Pharmacology

The effects of decentralisation and stimulation on the intact vas deferens were studied in vitro. Control and experimental vasa deferentia from the same animal were set up in parallel organ baths, and their responses to transmural nerve or muscle stimulation and applied noradrenaline were tested.

Results

Effect of Stimulation or Decentralisation in the Intact Vas Deferens

Table 1 compares the responses of experimental and control contralateral vasa deferentia to transmural stimulation in vitro following various periods of decentralisation or chronic preganglionic nerve stimulation. Contractures in response to repetitive electrical stimuli of 0.2 or 0.4 ms duration were recorded, all measurements being made at maximal stimulus strength and frequency (usually 80 v and 40 Hz). As Table 1 shows, decentralisation had little effect on the latency or contrac-

Table 1. Comparison between stimulated or decentralised vasa deferentia and control contralateral vasa deferentia

Days after operation	Latency (ms)		½ contraction time (ms)		Fatigability (% decrease)	
	Con.	Expt.	Con.	Expt.	Con.	Expt.
Decentralised						
7–14 days ($n=6$)	471 ± 75	475 ± 45	466 ± 87	442 ± 86	19 ± 12	32 ± 16
15–27 days ($n=3$)	460 ± 57	450 ± 50	533 ± 57	450 ± 50	32 ± 4	57 ± 1
Stimulated						
3–5 days ($n=4$)	432 ± 80	352 ± 46	500 ± 95	410 ± 81	26 ± 78	29 ± 10
6–8 days ($n=6$)	438 ± 41	340 ± 54	480 ± 95	330 ± 48	33 ± 14	31 ± 12

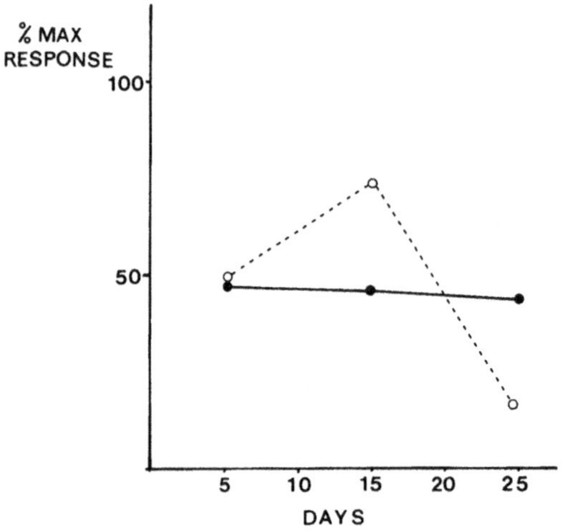

Fig. 1. Responses of decentralised vas deferens (○) compared with control contralateral vas deferens (●) to the concentration of noradrenaline (5×10^{-6} g/ml) at the mid-point of the concentration response curve expressed as % maximum response. Responses are shown at different times after decentralisation

tion time over the period examined, but there was a noticeable effect on fatigability (percentage decrease of the last of five consecutive contractions).

Although the time over which stimulated preparations could be examined was necessarily short, very large differences in latency and contraction time were seen compared with control contralateral vasa deferentia. Stimulation had little or no effect on fatigability.

Responses to Noradrenaline

One way of testing both the chemosensitivity and synaptic efficiency in the vas deferens is to measure the in vitro response to applied noradrenaline. Concentration response curves obtained from experimental vasa deferentia were compared with contralateral controls. Five days following decentralisation there was no difference between control and experimental preparations. By 15 days, decentralised prepara-

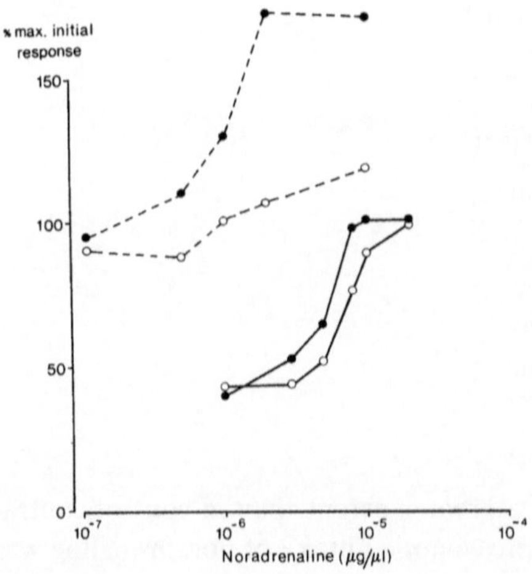

Fig. 2. Concentration-response curves to bath applied noradrenaline for control (●) and 7-day decentralised (○) vas deferens before *(unbroken lines)* and after *(broken lines)* 1×10^{-6} g/ml cocaine was added to the solution in the organ bath

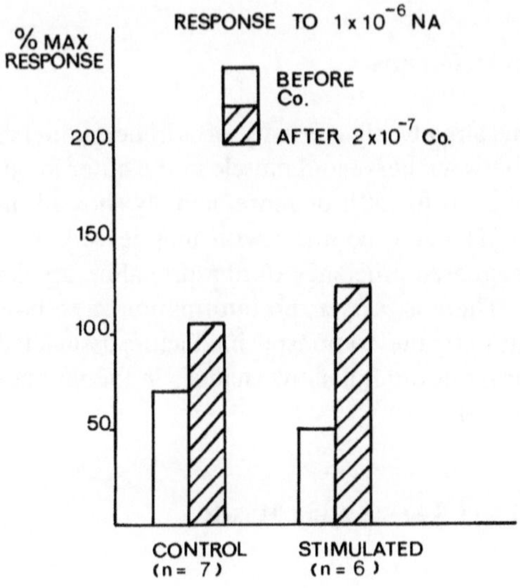

Fig. 3. Pooled responses of control and stimulated vasa deferentia to 1×10^{-6} noradrenaline before and after addition of cocaine *(Co)* to the bathing solution expressed as maximum response before the addition of the uptake inhibitor

tions showed slightly higher sensitivity to noradrenaline, while at 25 days they were less sensitive than controls (see Fig. 1). Differences in sensitivity to noradrenaline between control and decentralised preparations were not great, but responses obtained in the presence of cocaine or pertofran, which inhibit uptake of noradrenaline showed much greater differences. In the example shown in Fig. 2 the increase in sensitivity shown as a shift in the concentration response curve to noradrenaline in the presence of 1×10^{-6} mg/ml cocaine is less in a 7-day decentralised vas deferens than in the contralateral control from the same animal, indicating that decentralisation has an early influence reducing the uptake of noradrenaline by nerve varicosities.

Stimulation resulted in a small reduction in sensitivity to applied noradrenaline in most preparations but had a more dramatic effect on the noradrenaline uptake mechanism as is shown in Fig. 3. Responses to 1×10^{-6} mg/ml noradrenaline in prep-

Table 2. Total nerve profiles and close contacts per 100 muscle cells in intact stimulated vas deferens

Stimulation time		Total nerve profiles		Contacts within 100 n*M*	
Days	Hours	Con.	Stim.	Con.	Stim.
5	24	28	26	10	9
6	32	25	26	10	7
8	50	37	35	11	13
8	51	39	38	11	16

arations stimulated for 4 days increased to a greater extent than in control contralateral vasa deferentia, suggesting that the presynaptic uptake of noradrenaline was more efficient following stimulation.

Nerve Density in Intact Stimulated Vasa Deferentia

It is interesting to note that despite the already high density of adrenergic nerve varicosities and frequent close contacts between nerve and muscle in the outer longitudinal muscle layer, preparations stimulated for 50 h or more actually showed increased numbers of close (within 100 n*M*) nerve contacts with muscle cells (see Table 2). This could explain both the increased efficiency of noradrenaline uptake and the decreased latency of responses. There is, as yet, no information as to how long this effect lasts, but it is not thought to be due to nonspecific factors associated with surgery since sham operated preparations did not show changes in the number of close nerve/muscle contacts (Jones et al. 1983b).

Nerve Regeneration and Synaptic Density in Regenerating Muscle

Decentralisation

No changes in the total number of nerve profiles or close contacts were seen in decentralised intact vasa deferentia during the first 6 weeks. However, when reinnervation of minced regenerating muscle in animals with intact preganglionic pathways (referred to here as control animals) was compared with that seen after decentralisation clear differences emerge. While there is a steady increase in the total number of adrenergic nerve profiles per 100 muscle cells in both decentralised and control animals, the number of close contacts (within 100 nm of the nearest muscle cell) does not increase in step with the total nerve count after decentralisation. As Fig. 4 shows there is, if anything, a decrease with time in the number of close contacts during reinnervation of the decentralised vas deferens. In animals in which preganglionic pathways remain intact, the proportion of close contacts to total number of nerve profiles remains relatively constant throughout the reinnervation period,

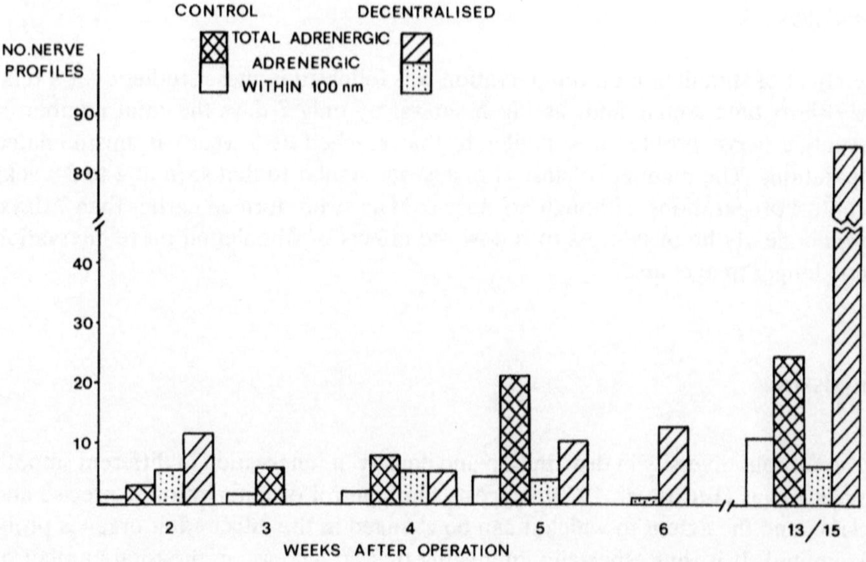

Fig. 4. The total number of nerve profiles and close contacts (within 100 n*M*) per 100 muscle cells in a minced regenerating portion of vas deferens at different times after operation. Reinnervation with adrenergic nerves with intact preganglionic pathways is compared with decentralised preparation

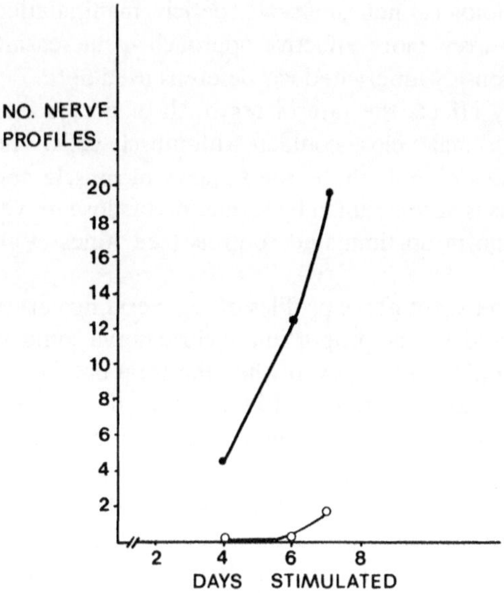

Fig. 5. Number of total adrenergic nerve profiles and close nerve-muscle contacts in minced regenerating vas deferens stimulated for different periods of time after operation

both reaching control values by 5 weeks, and slightly exceeding them at 13 to 15 weeks. In the decentralised preparations a great increase in the total number of nerves was seen at 13 weeks, the time when ganglionic cells become cholinergically reinnervated (Yokota and Burnstock 1983). However, this did not result in a proportional increase in the number of close contacts (see Fig. 4).

Stimulation

The effect of stimulation on reinnervation was followed in these studies over a relatively short time course and, as Fig. 5 shows, by only 7 days the total number of adrenergic nerve profiles was similar to that reached at 5 weeks in unstimulated preparations. The number of close contacts was similar to that seen at 2 to 3 weeks in control preparations, although no close contacts were formed earlier than 7 days. It would clearly be of interest to follow the effects of stimulation on reinnervation over a longer time course.

Discussion

The enormous diversity in distribution and density of innervation in different smooth muscle organs (Burnstock 1970) suggests that control of innervation is precise and specific, and the extent to which it can be changed in the intact adult organ is probably limited. It is thus especially interesting that an increase in the total number of close contacts between nerve and muscle can be induced by preganglionic nerve stimulation in the intact adult vas deferens. This is reflected in increased efficiency of neuromuscular responses, seen as reduced latency of the response to in vitro stimulation and enhanced transmitter uptake. In less densely innervated smooth muscle organs, or in those with a pathological neuromuscular deficit, manipulation of preganglionic pathways may be an even more effective approach to increasing neuromuscular efficiency than in the densely innervated vas deferens used here.

Preganglionic nerve activity clearly affects the rate of regrowth of nerves into regenerating muscle, and their ability to make close contacts with muscle cells. The relatively high number of nerve profiles seen at the earliest stages of muscle and nerve regeneration in stimulted animals is accompanied by formation of close nerve-muscle contacts at an earlier stage than in unstimulated controls (see Jones et al. 1983a).

A similar restoration in the total number of nerve profiles of regenerating nerves from decentralised ganglia did not form the same proportion of close nerve contacts as either control or stimulated regenerating nerves, even when the total number of nerve profiles greatly exceeded control values. The most likely explanation for this would seem to be that efficient transmitter release and uptake are required for the formation of close nerve-muscle contacts and the induction of post synaptic specialisation. A reduction in the ability of adrenergic nerve varicosities to take up noradrenaline is seen soon after decentralisation and presumably lasts throughout the period of decentralisation. During this time synaptic sites on decentralised ganglion cells are occupied by adrenergic nerve terminals until approximately 12 weeks after operation when cholinergic innervation is re-established (Yokota and Burnstock 1983). It would appear that during this time, although adrenergic nerves can grow, sprouting profusely throughout the minced regenerating muscle cells, and probably within the ganglia too, they are unable to establish synaptic contacts with the regenerating muscle cells. Whether this is solely due to a lack of transganglionic neural activity, or whether other factors are involved is not clear. Noradrenaline content and uptake were not studied in the long-term decentralised, but intact, vasa deferentia, but it would be interesting to see whether the ability of nerves to form close contacts with regenerating muscle was indeed related to restoration of normal noradrenaline uptake and storage. One final point to be considered is that if nerve terminal arborisation is increased, as it appears to be in long-term decentralised preparations undergoing regeneration, but neurones are synthesising transmitter at a reduced rate, the amount of transmitter available at release sites will remain low. Thus, to achieve reinnervation, conditions promoting nerve sprouting must be tempered with maintenance of a high level of transmitter production.

References

Black IB, Bloom EM, Hamill RW (1976) Central regulation of sympathetic neuron development. Proc Natl Acad Sci USA 73:3575–3578

Bloom EM, Hamill RW, Black IB (1976) Elevation of tyrosine hydroxylase activity in sympathetic neurons after reserpine: the role of the central nervous system. Brain Res 115:525–528

Burnstock G (1970) Structure of smooth muscle and its innervation. In: Bullbring E, Brading A, Jones A, Tomita T (eds) Smooth muscle. Arnold, London, pp 1–69

Burnstock G, Dennison M, Jones R (1978a) Chronic stimulation of the hypogastric nerve in the male guinea-pig in vivo. J Physiol 276:2–3P

Burnstock G, Yokota R, Jones R (1978b) Reinnervation of regenerating smooth muscle cells in minced vas deferens of the guinea-pig. Cell Tissue Res 190:495–508

Furness JB, Iwayama T (1972) The arrangement and identification of axons innervating the vas deferens of the guinea-pig. J Anat 113:179–196

Gillespie JS, McGrath JC (1974) The effect of pithing and of nerve stimulation on the depletion of noradrenaline by reserpine in the rat anoccygeus muscle and vas deferens. Br J Pharmacol 52:585–590

Jones R, Yokota R, Burnstock G (1983a) The long term influence of decentralisation or preganglionic hypogastric nerve stimulation in vivo on the reinnervation of minced vas deferens in the guinea-pig. Cell Tissue Res 232:281–293

Jones R, Dennison ME, Burnstock G (1983b) The effect of decentralisation or chronic nerve stimulation in vivo on the innervation and responses of the guinea-pig vas deferens. Cell Tissue Res 232:265–279

Saito A, Kasuya Y, Goto K (1981) The role of morphological and functional changes in adrenergic nerves for the development of colchicine-induced supersensitivity in the rat vas deferens. J Pharmacol Exp Ther 217:516–523

Thoenen H (1972) Comparison between the effect of neuronal activity and nerve growth factor on the enzymes involved in the synthesis of norepinephrine. Pharmacol Rev 24:255–267

Tranzer JP, Thoenen H (1967) Electronmicroscopic localisation of 5-hydroxdopamine (3,4,5,-trihydroxyphenylethylamine) a new "false" sympathetic transmitter. Experientia 32:743–745

Yokota R, Burnstock G (1983) Decentralisation of neurones in the pelvic ganglion of the guinea-pig: reinnervation by adrenergic nerves. Cell Tissue Res 232:399–411

Yokota R, Burnstock G, Jones R, Brown MD (1978) An ultrastructural study of regeneration of minced smooth muscle in the vas deferens of the guinea-pig. Cell Tissue Res 190:481–493

Zigmond RE, Chalazonitis A (1979) Long term effects of preganglionic nerve stimulation on tyrosine hydroxylase activity in the rat superior cervical ganglion. Brain Res 164:137–152

III. Muscle Plasticity in Disease

The Role of Passive Stretch in Retarding Muscle Atrophy*

D. F. Goldspink[1] and G. Goldspink[2,3]

Introduction

The skeletal musculature comprises the largest single tissue of the body, contributing up to 40%–45% of the adult body weight and 75% of its protein mass (Goldspink et al. 1985). Clearly this means that muscle is extremely important to the organism in metabolic terms, in addition to its well recognized mechanical functions of locomotion and maintenance of posture. Like many other tissues of the body, skeletal muscle undergoes atrophy in response to the loss of functional demands. In contrast, rapid adaptive growth can be induced either by the subsequent return of these functions or by the imposition of new, greater work demands. This plasticity (Pette 1980) represents part of the overall biological economy of the body in maintaining, or withdrawing, structures according to the changing requirements of the organism. Such features are regularly observed clinically; situations of disuse producing muscle wasting and weakness, while compensatory growth of the relevant musculature is often linked to patient recovery and rehabilitation.

Muscle disuse can arise in a variety of ways, e.g. from the immobilization of joints through disease or injury (Young et al. 1982), after cerebral or spinal cord damage, tenotomy (Goldspink et al. 1983), denervation (Gutmann 1962), or weightlessness. The latter situation can be wide ranging, from simple bed rest resulting from debilitating illnesses to the loss of gravity and postural activities during space travel (Feller et al. 1981). In all of these examples the normally highly active (Fischback and Robbins 1969; Hnik et al. 1985) antigravity muscles, such as the soleus, are more profoundly affected by disuse (Goldspink 1980). Such slow-twitch muscles exhibit a rapid and extensive atrophy in response to the deprivation of normal activity patterns (see below). Changes in the size and strength of skeletal muscle also have wider implications. Normal muscle function has an important bearing on the growth, or atrophy, of other components within the musculoskeletal system, such as tendons, ligaments and bone. For example the cortical thickness and degree of mineralisation of bone is believed to be dependent, at least in part, upon the mechanical stresses normally imposed on the skeleton by the musculature. Hence, muscle inactivity induces atrophy in both muscle and the skeleton (Morey and Baylink 1978). Obtaining

---

* This work was supported by a grant from NASA-Ames No. NAG 2-272 and the Wellcome Trust to G. Goldspink, D. F. Goldspink was the recipient of a Wellcome Trust travel award

1 Department of Physiology, The Queen's University of Belfast, Medical Biology Centre, 97 Lisburn Road, Belfast, BT9 7BL, Northern Ireland, U.K.

2 Department of Anatomy & Cellular Biology, School of Medicine, Tuft's University, 136 Harrison Avenue, Boston, Massachusetts 02111, U.S.A.

3 Present address: Department of Cell Biology, Royal Veterinary College, London

Electrical Stimulation and Neuromuscular Disorders
Ed. by W. A. Nix and G. Vrbová

a clearer understanding of the cellular basis of muscle atrophy would therefore represent an important step in attempting to prevent, or retard, wasting within the musculoskeletal system, and in countering secondary changes (e.g. the accumulation of connective tissue and the resultant muscle inextensibility) which can hinder patient rehabilitation.

One experimental system designed to render muscles less active will now be described in more detail. The ensuing muscle atrophy will be explained by consideration of the crucial changes in the rates of protein turnover.

Muscle Atrophy Arising from Hypokinesia and Hypodynamia

A number of experimental models have been employed to simulate the weightless state, as experienced in space. One such animal model recently employed by us (i.e. in collaboration with Paul Loughna and Alison Morton) was a suspension method, similar to that described by Musacchia et al. (1980). Rats (initially weighing 100 g) were individually placed in a cloth harness designed to fit snugly around the torso while allowing the four limbs to project through appropriate openings in the harness. The restrained animal was then suspended by the harness from a metal bar located at the top of each cage (Fig. 1). This procedure allows the two forelimbs to rest on a metal tray, so positioned to provide the rat with free continuous access to food and water. In contrast, the animal's hind limbs were completely unsupported and therefore devoid of all normal weight bearing, or force producing, functions (i.e. hypodynamia). Within a few hours these suspended animals rarely moved their hind limbs (i.e. hypokinesia), leaving them to hang freely in space. The effects of this combined hypokinesia and hypodynamia on the hind limb musculature was studied as a function of time. Although the suspended rats had unrestricted access to food, they ate approximately 20% less than fully mobile, ad libitum fed animals. Since protein turnover, and hence growth, of skeletal muscle is sensitive to dietary supply (Waterlow et al. 1978), such differences in food intake were taken into account in order to study muscle inactivity in isolation of such dietary considerations. Nutritionally matched control rats were therefore pair fed to the same daily intake as the suspended animals.

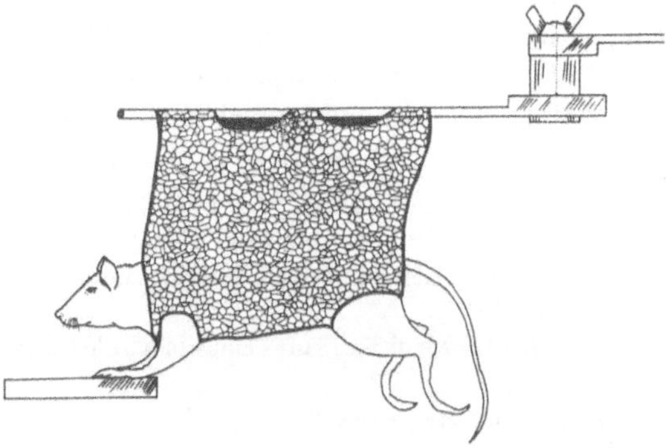

Fig. 1. A suspension model designed to induce a state of hypokinesia and hypodynamia in the hind limb muscles. In such suspended animals force production is reduced (hypodynamia) and muscle contraction greatly decreased (hypokinesia) in the hind limbs

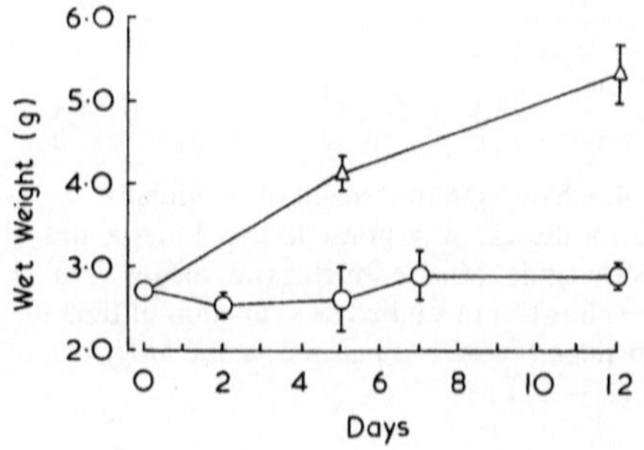

Fig. 2. Changes in the weight of the hind limb musculature under simulated weightless conditions. The wet weight of all muscles in one hind limb of suspended (○—○) or pair fed, ambulatory control (△—△) rats was measured as a function of time. Each value represents the mean ± SEM of measurements on legs from at least 5 animals in each group

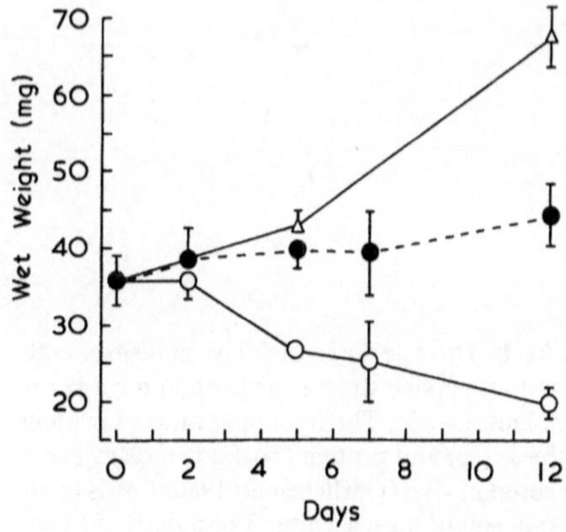

Fig. 3. Changes in the weight of the soleus muscle in response to hypokinesia and hypodynamia, with or without passive stretching. The slow-twitch soleus muscle in suspended rats was weighed in both free hanging (○—○) or dorsiflexed immobilized (●----●) limbs. The weights (means ± SEM) of these muscles from a minimum of six limbs were compared with those taken from pair fed, ambulatory controls (△—△)

The simulated weightless state induced marked differences in the whole musculature of the hind limb, as compared with that of the pair fed controls (Fig. 2). While no true atrophy occurred over the 12 days studied, the muscles of the hind limb failed to grow (i.e. at only 0.6% per day) in these suspended animals. This contrasted with a growth rate of approximately 5.5% per day in the musculature of the control animals (Fig. 2). As elsewhere in the body, the musculature of the hind limb is composed of different muscle types, possessing varying proportions of slow- (i.e. slow-oxidative) and fast- (fast glycolytic and fast-oxidative glycolytic) twitch fibres. Consequently, several individual muscles of the lower hind limb were examined under the same conditions. A distinctive order of responsiveness to the 12 days of disuse emerged, with wasting of the soleus > gastrocnemius > plantaris > extensor digitorum longus and tibialis anterior.

More detailed information will now be presented for the two muscles exhibiting the most extreme responses, i.e. the soleus (Fig. 3) and tibialis anterior (Fig. 4). Decreased activity in the soleus was accompanied by a rapid and sustained true atrophy (Fig. 3). In contrast, disuse induced much smaller losses of weight and intracellular protein from the fast-twitch muscle at all of the times studied (Fig. 4). In addition in the tibialis anterior, but not the soleus, there were signs of renewed growth from 5 days of hypokinesia and hypodynamia onwards (Figs. 3 and 4).

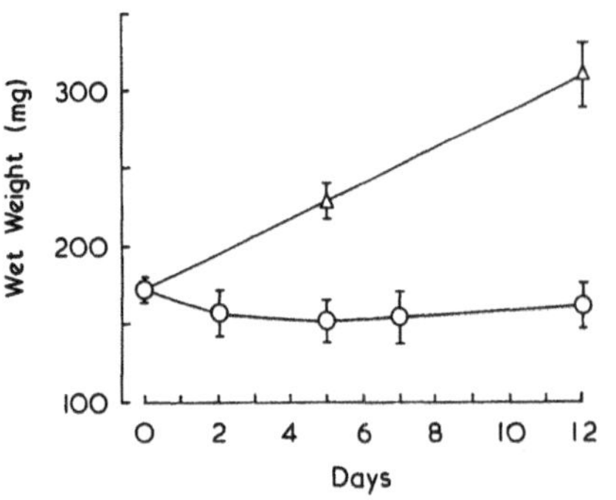

Fig. 4. Changes in the weight of the tibialis anterior muscle in response to hypokinesia and hypodynamia. Muscle weights (i.e. means ± SEM of 6 values) were studied as a function of time in suspended (O—O) or pair fed, ambulatory control (Δ—Δ) rats

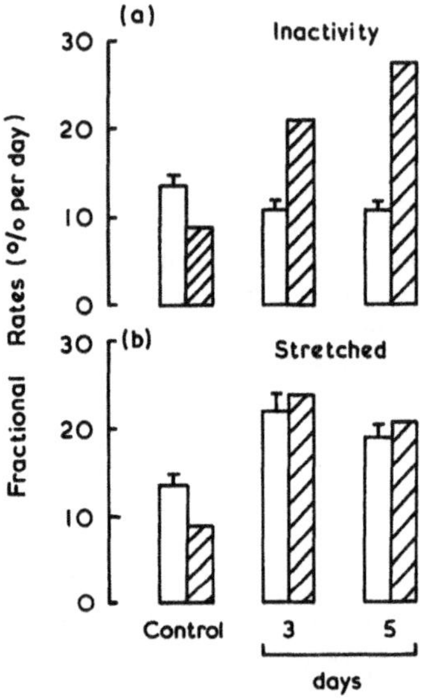

Fig. 5a, b. The effect of 3 or 5 days of disuse, with or without passive stretch, on protein turnover in the soleus muscle. The fractional rates of protein synthesis (□) and protein breakdown (▨) were measured in vivo (Garlick et al. 1980; Lewis et al. 1984) in soleus muscles after 3 or 5 days of hypokinesia and hypodynamia, with (**b**) or without (**a**) permanent stretching by immobilization in dorsiflexion. Each value is the mean ± SEM of measurements made on a minimum of 6 muscles in each group

Changes in Protein Turnover with Disuse

Intracellular protein is of course the largest nonaqueous component of muscle, representing approximately 20% of the tissue wet weight at this animal age (Lewis et al. 1984). Muscle growth (i.e. protein accretion) or atrophy (i.e. protein depletion) must therefore be regulated by changes in the relative rates of protein synthesis and protein degradation. Hence, to gain a fuller understanding of these alterations in muscle size it is necessary to establish what, if any, changes had been induced in these two regulatory processes. Rates of protein synthesis and breakdown were therefore measured in vivo by the best available techniques using ^{3}H-phenylalanine as the tracer amino acid (Garlick et al. 1980; Lewis et al. 1984). In order to gain insight into the early events responsible for the muscle atrophy (Figs. 3 and 4), protein turnover was measured in both the soleus (Fig. 5) and tibialis anterior (Fig. 6) muscles of control and suspended animals 3 and 5 days after commencing the study.

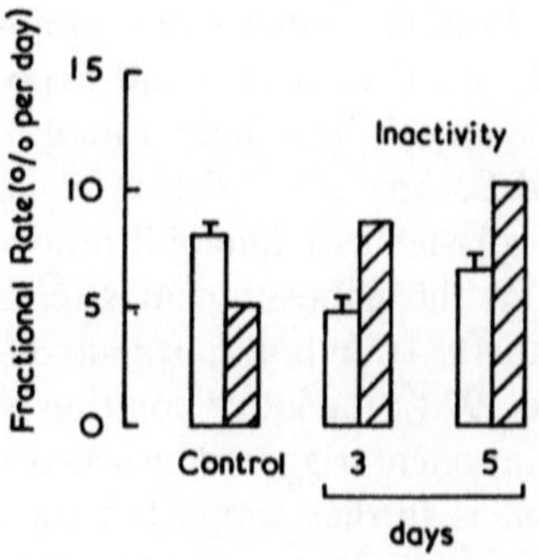

Fig. 6. The effects of 3 or 5 days of hypokinesia and hypodynamia on protein turnover in the tibialis anterior muscle. The fractional rates of protein synthesis (□) and protein degradation (■) were measured in the tibialis anterior after 3 or 5 days of disuse, as induced by the suspension model (Fig. 1). These muscles were taken from the same animals as in Fig. 5

The wasting of the antigravity soleus muscle was explained by a significant decrease in the fractional rate of synthesis (i.e. the fraction of the protein mass synthesized per day) and a large increase in the rate of breakdown after 3 or 5 days of hypokinesia and hypodynamia (Fig. 5a). Similar events were also found in the tibialis anterior (Fig. 6). However, like the degree of atrophy, changes in protein turnover were more pronounced in the soleus than in the tibialis muscle. Similar observations have also been made when fast and slow muscles have been rendered considerably less active (Fischbach and Robbins 1969; Hnik et al. 1985) by immobilization in either a partially or fully shortened position (Goldspink 1980). Another feature consistent with previous studies (Waterlow et al. 1978; Lewis et al. 1984) is the higher basal rates of protein synthesis and breakdown in the slow-twitch muscle (Fig. 5a), compared with fast-twitch muscles (Fig. 6; note the expanded scale in this figure).

The Role of Stretch in Preventing Disuse Atrophy

When hypokinesia and hypodynamia were imposed on muscles which were permanently stretched a different series of events was observed. In this instance the ankle of one hind limb of the suspended rats was immobilized throughout in a dorsiflexed position (using strong tape). This form of immobilization holds the soleus muscle in a lengthened, stretched state (Williams and Goldspink 1973). Under these conditions no true atrophy occurred with hypokinesia and hypodynamia (Fig. 3). Rather the stretched muscle grew, albeit more slowly than the control. In some other experimental models in animals (Goldspink 1980) and birds (Holly et al. 1980) additional growth, beyond that of the controls, has been observed. In these cases the stretched muscles increase their girth (Holly et al. 1980) and length, the latter being accomplished by the addition of new sarcomeres in series (Williams and Goldspink 1973). It is clear, therefore, that passive stretch is effective in preventing muscle atrophy despite the deprivation of normal activity patterns.

Stretch-Induced Changes in Protein Turnover

Stretching the soleus muscle for 3 or 5 days produced marked changes in protein turnover, both with respect to nonstretched soleus muscles in ambulatory control and suspended (free, unrestrained limb) rats (Fig. 5b). Protein synthesis was significantly increased, i.e. a reversal of the changes found with hypokinesia and hypodynamia alone (Fig. 5a). Similar increases in protein synthesis have been found in stretched muscles when measured in vivo (Booth and Seider 1979; Watson et al. 1984) or in vitro (Goldspink 1977) after appropriate plaster cast immobilization. Such changes have been detected as early as 6h after the imposition of stretch (Goldspink 1977; Booth and Seider 1979; Watson et al. 1984), in both normally innervated and denervated muscles (Goldspink 1977 and 1978); the latter pointing to a passive, myogenic response rather than any active component triggered by sensory receptors within the stretched soleus. This conclusion is further supported by a recent EMG study (Hnik et al. 1985) in which no enhanced discharge was found from chronically stretched muscles. In addition to the enhancement of protein synthesis, the rate of degradation was also increased in the stretched soleus, leading to higher turnover rates in this muscle, compared with its control (Fig. 5b). Although the rate of protein breakdown has also been found to change upon stretching isolated muscles in vitro (Goldberg et al. 1975; Etlinger et al. 1981), the changes described in such isolated preparation have often been of a variable nature. This variability can to some extent be explained by differences in the initial length of the isolated muscles (i.e. prior to stretching) relative to their resting lengths in vivo (Etlinger et al. 1981).

Unfortunately, it is difficult to isolate with certainty the influences of stretch from other variables, e.g. reduced activity, in such systems. Nonetheless, it would seem probable that the increased rate of protein synthesis represents a genuine influence of stretch, the mechanical stresses imposed on the muscle membranes somehow stimulating the production of prostaglandins, which have been shown to enhance protein turnover (Rodemann and Goldberg 1982; Palmer et al. 1983). Since protein breakdown is increased, whether a muscle is stretched (Fig. 5b) or held in a shortened disused state (Fig. 5a; Goldspink 1977), the changes in degradation may simply reflect the reduced activity at both muscle lengths (Hnik et al. 1985).

Unfortunately, the therapeutic applications of stretch may be limited. Its growth-promoting effects on an individual muscle (e.g. the soleus) or a group of functional synergists are likely to be accompanied by adverse effects on antagonist muscles (e.g. tibialis anterior). Such antagonists would probably be restrained in a shortened position, and this would induce muscle wasting (Williams and Goldspink 1973; Goldspink 1980). This type of effect can be observed in patients who have suffered a stroke. Some muscles in paraplegic limbs become visably enlarged while others show extensive wastage, this depending upon the position the limb joint is restrained in. Intermittent, rather than permanent, stretching is, however, likely to be beneficial in rehabilitating patients. However, the critical amount of stretch and the duration of its imposition to produce maximal effects remain ill-defined.

Electrical Stimulation

The fibre type composition, and hence the metabolic and contractile characteristics, of a muscle change throughout much of postnatal life (Buller et al. 1960a; Goldspink and Ward 1979). The age-related decline in the rate of protein turnover is probably linked to the slowing down of such cellular differentiation upon progressing towards old age (Lewis et al. 1984). Despite these developmental changes, gene expression can still be influenced by a variety of physiological factors, which by modifying the transcription and translation of specific proteins can change the muscle's morphological, metabolic and functional characteristics. Hence, in addition to the genetic endowment other factors, such as hormones (Ianuzzo et al. 1977), diet (C. Boreham, B.J. Merry, P.E. Williams, G. Goldspink and D.F. Goldspink – unpublished information), exercise (Costill et al. 1976; Watt et al. 1982) and experimentally-induced changes in neuronal activity (Salmons and Henriksson 1981; Pette 1984) can influence fibre type composition, as well as muscle size and mechanical strength.

The now classical experiments of Buller et al. (1960b) first indicated the importance of the nerve supply in determining the contractile characteristics of different muscle types; the cross-innervation of fast and slow muscles led to the reversal of their normal twitch characteristics. Similar transformations of fast- to slow-twitch muscles have subsequently been achieved by superimposing frequency patterns which are usually delivered only to slow muscles (i.e. 5–10 Hz) onto the normal (fast) nerve supply (Salmons and Vrbová 1969). Since these early experiments numerous studies have been undertaken to determine the effects of chronic stimulation on muscle metabolism and function. These studies have demonstrated a series of intermediate steps which help to explain the transformations in contractile characteristics at both cellular and molecular levels (see Salmons and Henriksson 1981; Pette 1984). Although many of these chronically stimulated muscles do become smaller in size, continuous stimulation of rabbit muscles over 14 days has recently been shown to prevent the muscle wasting which normally accompanies immobilization in a partially shortened state (Cotter and Phillips 1985).

Electrical Stimulation Coupled with Stretch

Preliminary studies (in collaboration with Pamela Williams) have also shown that potentially beneficial therepeutic effects can be obtained by combining passive stretch and electrical stimulation over shorter time periods. Although only data for the extensor digitorum longus muscle (a fast muscle like the tibialis anterior) are presented here, similar trends were observed in other muscles, including the slow soleus muscle. In this particular experiment the extensor digitorum longus muscle of one hind leg of adult rabbits was permanently stretched (via plaster cast immobilization) for 5 days, with or without continuous stimulation (at 5 Hz) via electrodes positioned close to the sciatic nerve in the thigh. Contralateral (sham-operated) limb muscles were used as control tissues in each experimental system. The animals were killed after 5 days of treatment and 15 min after receiving an intravenous injection of 150 µmol ^{3}H-phenylalanine per 100 g body weight (Garlick et al. 1980). The excised muscles were rapidly sectioned into five equal lengths passing from one tendon to the other. Each region was frozen in liquid nitrogen and subsequently analyzed to determine the fractional rates of protein synthesis (Garlick et al. 1980).

Regionalized Changes in Protein Synthesis in Response to Stretch and Electrical Stimulation

Stretch alone caused a 24% increase in the whole muscle weight and approximately 13% increase in its length. As in the case of rat muscles (Fig. 5b), this stretch-induced growth was accompanied by increased rates of protein synthesis. However, in the much larger rabbit muscles it was possible to establish that this stimulation of synthesis was located along the entire length of the stretched muscle (Fig. 7). Changes in the synthetic rates in the end regions (i.e. 1 and 5) are consistent with earlier reports describing longitudinal growth of myofibrils through the serial addition of new sarcomeres (Williams and Goldspink 1973). The enhancement of synthetic rates in the more centrally-located regions (i.e. 2–4) is also in keeping with the fibre hypertrophy which is known to occur in stretched muscles (Holly et al. 1980).

The combination of stretch and electrical stimulation for 5 days resulted in even greater increases in the synthetic rates in the central, but not end, regions of the muscle. Although no equivalent measurements on the rates of protein breakdown were possible at the time, these massive increases in synthesis were reflected in 21% and 15% increases in the weight and length of the stretched, stimulated muscle, when compared with contralateral controls. At this stage we are not in a position to distinguish between the type of proteins being synthesized; hence, we do not know whether there is any selective synthesis of one type of protein over another, and if this varies in the different regions along the length of the muscle. More experiments are underway to define more clearly the time scale of these changes, and to optimize

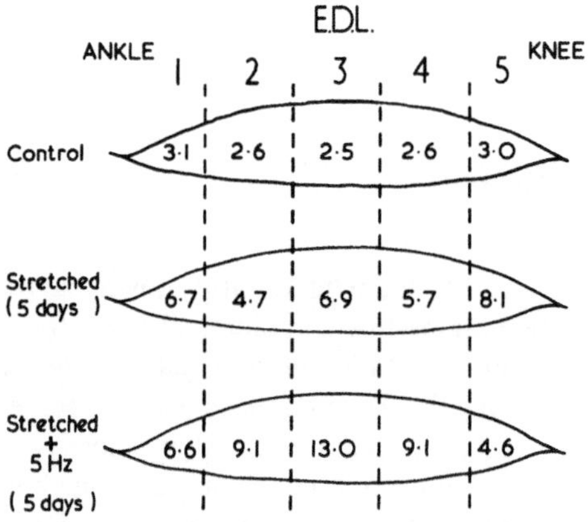

Fig. 7. Regionalized changes in protein synthesis in the extensor digitorum longus after 5 days of stretch or combined stretch and electrical stimulation. One hind limb of rabbits was immobilized in plantar flexion (Williams and Goldspink 1973) for 5 days to stretch the extensor digitorum longus muscle. In other animals the same procedure was combined with continuous electrical stimulation (5 Hz) via implanted electrodes positioned close to the sciatic nerve. Contralateral limb muscles were used as controls in all cases. All rabbits were injected with ^{3}H-phenylalanine 15 min prior to being killed, in order to measure protein synthesis in these muscles (Garlick et al. 1980). The fractional rates of protein synthesis (% per day; i.e. the percentage of the protein mass synthesized per day) in each of the 5 regions are shown above. It is clear that stretch, with or without simultaneous stimulation, enhanced synthetic rates in this muscle

the frequency and duration of stimulation in conjunction with stretching. Clearly the combination of passive stretch and electrical stimulation may prove to be a useful therapeutic tool This may be especially so since we, like Cotter and Phillips (1985), found that the stimulated antagonists (i.e. held in a shortened state) underwent very little atrophy compared with situations where these muscles were simply immobilized in this position without any stimulation (Goldspink 1980).

References

Booth FW, Seider MJ (1979) Early changes in skeletal muscle protein synthesis after immobilization of rats. J Appl Physiol 47:974–977

Buller AJ, Eccles JC, Eccles RM (1960a) Differentiation of fast and slow muscles in the cat hind limb. J Physiol (Lond) 150:399–416

Buller AJ, Eccles JC, Eccles RM (1960b) Interactions between motor neurones and muscles in respect of the characteristic speeds of their responses. J Physiol (Lond) 150:417–439

Costill DL, Daniels J, Evans W, Fink W, Krahenbuhl G, Saltin B (1976) Skeletal muscle enzymes and fiber composition in male and female track athletes. J Appl Physiol 40:149–154

Cotter M, Phillips P (1985) Chronic low-frequency activation prevents immobilization atrophy in rabbit soleus muscles. J Physiol (Lond) 361:35P

Etlinger JD, Kameyama T, Van der Westhuysen D, Erlij D, Matsumoto K (1981) In: Guba F, Marechal G, Takacs O (eds) Mechanisms of muscle adaptation to functional requirements. Pergamon, New York, pp 241–253

Feller DD, Ginoza HS, Morey ER (1981) Atrophy of rat skeletal muscles in stimulated weightlessness. Physiologist 24:S9–10

Fischback GD, Robbins N (1969) Changes in contractile properties of disused soleus muscles. J Physiol 201:305–320

Garlick PJ, McNurlan MA, Preedy VR (1980) A rapid and convenient technique for measuring the rate of protein synthesis in tissues by injection of [^{3}H] phenylalanine. Biochem J 192:719–723

Goldberg AL, Etlinger JD, Goldspink DF, Jablecki C (1975) Mechanism of work-induced hypertrophy of skeletal muscle. Med Sci Sports 7:248–261

Goldspink DF (1977) The influence of immobilization and stretch on protein turnover of rat skeletal muscle. J Physiol 264:267–282

Goldspink DF (1978) The influence of passive stretch on the growth and protein turnover of the denervated EDL muscle. Biochem J 174:595–602

Goldspink DF (1980) The influence of contractile activity and the nerve supply on muscle size and protein turnover. In: Pette D (ed) Plasticity of muscle. Walter de Gruyter, Berlin, pp 525–539

Goldspink G, Ward PS (1979) Changes in rodent muscle fibre types during post-natal growth, undernutrition and exercise. J Physiol 296–453–469

Goldspink DF, Garlick PJ, McNurlan MA (1983) Protein turnover measured in vivo and in vitro in muscles undergoing compensatory growth and subsequent denervation atrophy. Biochem J 210:89–98

Goldspink DF, Lewis SEM, Kelly FJ (1985) Protein turnover and cathepsin B activity in several individual tissues of foetal and senescent rats. Comp Biochem Physiol 82:849–853

Gutmann E (ed) (1962) The denervated muscle. Czechoslovakian Academy of Science, Prague

Hnik P, Vejsada R, Goldspink, DF, Kasicki S, Krekule I (1985) Quantitative evaluation of EMG activity in rat extensor and flexor muscles immobilized at different lengths. Exp Neurol 88:515–528

Holly RG, Barnett JG, Ashmore CR, Taylor RG, Mole PA (1980) Stretch-induced growth in chicken wing muscles: a new model of stretch hypertrophy. Am J Physiol 238:C62–C71

Ianuzzo D, Patel P, Chen V, O'Brien P, Williams C (1977) Thyroidal trophic influence on skeletal muscle myosin. Nature 270:74–76

Lewis SEM, Kelly FJ, Goldspink DF (1984) Pre- and post-natal growth and protein turnover in smooth muscle, heart and slow- and fast-twitch skeletal muscles of the rat. Biochem J 217:517–526

Morey ER, Baylink DJ (1978) Inhibition of bone formation during space flight. Science 201:1138–1141

Musacchia XJ, Deavers DR, Meininger GA, Davis TP (1980) A model for hypokinesia: effects on muscle atrophy in the rat. J Appl Physiol 48:479–486

Palmer RM, Reeds PJ, Atkinson T, Smith RH (1983) The influence of changes in tension on protein synthesis and prostaglandin release in isolated rabbit muscles. Biochem J 214:1011–1014

Pette D (ed) (1980) Plasticity of muscle. Walter de Gruyter, Berlin

Pette D (1984) Activity-induced fast to slow transitions in mammalian muscle. Med Sci Sports Exerc 16:517–528

Rodemann HP, Goldberg AL (1982) Arachidonic acid, prostaglandin E_2 and $F_{2\alpha}$ influence rates of protein turnover in skeletal and cardiac muscle. J Biol Chem 257:1632–1638

Salmons S, Henriksson J (1981) The adaptive response of skeletal muscle to increased use. Muscle Nerve 4:94–105

Salmons S, Vrbová G (1969) The influence of activity on some contractile characteristics of mammalian fast and slow muscles. J Physiol (Lond) 210:535–549

Waterlow JC, Garlick PJ, Millward DJ (eds) (1978) The effects of nutrition and hormones on protein turnover in muscle. In: Protein turnover in mammalian tissues and in the whole body. North-Holland, Amsterdam, pp 625–696

Watson PA, Stein JP, Booth FW (1984) Changes in actin synthesis and actin-mRNA content in rat muscle during immobilization. Am J Physiol 247:C39–C44

Watt PW, Kelly FJ, Goldspink DF, Goldspink G (1982) Exercise-induced morphological and biochemical changes in skeletal muscles of the rat. J Appl Physiol 53:1144–1151

Williams PE, Goldspink G (1973) The effect of immobilization on the longitudinal growth of striated muscle. J Anat 116:45–55

Young A, Hughes I, Round JM, Edwards RHT (1982) The effect of knee injury on the number of muscle fibres in the human quadriceps femoris. Clin Sci 62:227–234

Stimulation of Denervated Muscle: What Do Isometric and Isotonic Recordings Tell Us?

D. M. Lewis[1], W. S. Al-Amood[1], and C. Rosendorff[2]

In recording the contractile (or dynamic) properties of muscle, two standard sets of conditions are commonly used. In one, the isometric set, the muscle is held at a constant length and the tension that develops is measured. The other, namely the isotonic set, involves allowing the muscle to shorten under constant load and recording changes of length. In the body, of course, muscle activity is more complex, sometimes involving periods approximating to isometric or isotonic, but more often shortening occurs under varying load. When lifting a weight, for example, arm muscles must first contract isometrically, developing sufficient tension to overcome the force of gravity on the weight (and on the arm). This will be followed by shortening but with the load on the muscles greater than in the isometric phase because additional force must be generated to accelerate the mass of the load (and of the arm). Only if a constant speed of movement is reached, will the shortening be truly isotonic. As the movement is ended and the arm is slowed, the inertia of the mass will exert a force in the opposite direction, which has to be opposed by action of antagonists. Finally, isometric contraction will hold the weight up. Natural contractions are also more complex than in experimental recordings because, as in the example described above, the activation of the muscle is not constant. A varying number of motor units are recruited, with changing discharge rates at different stages of the activity, according to the command signal from the brain and feedback from many receptors. Despite the complexity of natural activity, it is theoretically possible to analyse the resultant forces and movement in terms of muscle properties revealed by experimental isometric and isotonic recordings. Thus, the experimental conditions are chosen for reproductibility and easy interpretation.

Isometric Recordings

For isometric recordings the transducer used should ideally be infinitely stiff. In practice all instruments allow a small amount of shortening, which will normally be less than that permitted by tendons or the connexions made between muscle and transducer. The small shortening in the transducer is proportional to the force generated by the muscle. A simple version can be made from a metal bar fixed at one end and bent into a hook at the other to connect to the muscle (Fig. 1a, b). The displacement at the end of the bar is approximately equal to

$$4\,F\,l^2 / E\,w\,t^3$$

where F is the force applied; l, w and t are the length, width and thickness of the bar

1 Department of Physiology, University of Bristol, England
2 Department of Physiology, University of Witwatersrand, South Africa

Electrical Stimulation and Neuromuscular Disorders
Ed. by W. A. Nix and G. Vrbová

and E is Young's modulus of the material (i.e. its stiffness, e.g. $1.5 \times 10^5\,N/mm^2$ for steel).

The formula is only approximate since it is derived for a bar with a perfect rectangular shape. In addition to the need that the transducer should be stiff enough to minimise muscle shortening, it is also necessary that the bar should resonate at a sufficiently high frequency. If the frequency is too low, oscillations may distort the tension record. As a working rule, if the period of the cycle of the resonating bar is some 8–10 times shorter than the rising phase of the muscle twitch (the time to peak) then the response will be undistorted. The resonant frequency of a bar such as described above will be approximately $4\,t\,l^2/3$ MHz, but it is essential to test directly by setting the arm oscillating with a sudden change of force (e.g. burning through a thin thread supporting a weight). The frequency of oscillations can be measured and excessive damping (which would slow down the recording) detected by the oscillations falling away in less than 3 cycles.

Normally the tension-dependent bending of the bar will be monitored by strain gauges (Fig. 1a, b). Semiconductor gauges are normally used because of their high sensitivity. The fitting of our gauges for a Wheatstone's bridge often requires very small gauges, and one source of a wide range of shapes and sizes is Kulite Sensors.

It is best to use epoxy resins for bonding the gauges to the bar. Details of best materials have been described by Hodgson (1982) and Brooks (1984). Other types of transducer may be used to measure the tension-related length change, but semiconductor ones are the easiest to make for a particular task if commercial tension-transducers do not meet special requirements. Moreover, a sensible choice of commercial equipment can only be made if the problems of isometric recording are understood.

In optimising the design of a gauge for a specific task a compromise must be made between a device which is sensitive enough to give an adequate signal but stiff enough to prevent excessive shortening. Figure 2 illustrates the effects of deliberately introducing compliance into a recording system, in this experiment by record-

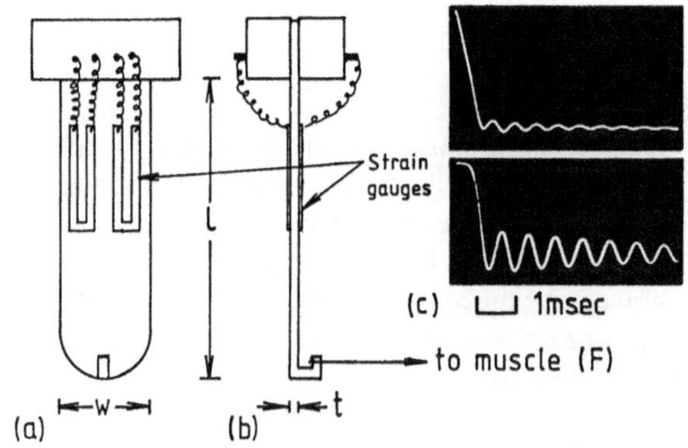

Fig. 1a–c. Isometric recording. **a, b** Front and side view of tension transducer, made from a flat bar with dimensions *(w, l, t)* described in the text. **c** Output of the strain gauge bridge in response to step change of tension applied to two transducers made of titanum in which w = 5 mm and 1 = 15 mm. *Above,* t = 0.8 mm and the force change was 5 N; *below,* t = 0.4 mm and force change 0.5 N. Note the difference between resonant frequencies (both recorded at same sweep speed)

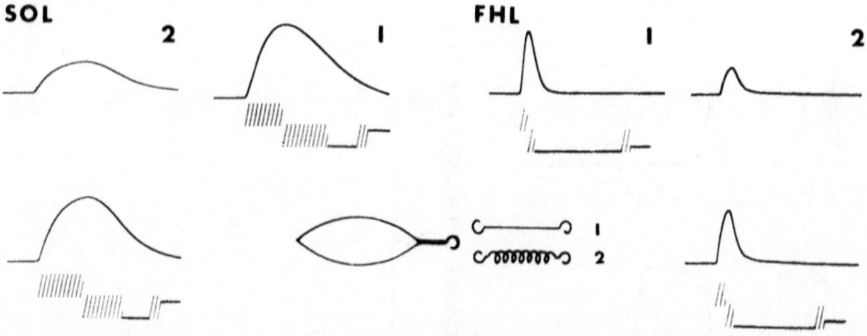

Fig. 2. Effects on isometric twitches of increasing the compliance in the recording system by inserting a flexible spring between the muscle and tension recorder (see inset diagram). Records from *FHL* (fast) and *SOL*eus (slow). In each case the true isometric twitch is shown under *1* and that recorded with extra compliance under *2* – *above* at the same amplification as 1 and *below* at 2.5 times higher gain. The series of *dots* under records indicate (i) time to peak in ms (raised set of dots), (ii) time to half relaxation, and (iii) peak active tension, where each dot is equivalent to 10 and 4 g force (approximately 100 or 40 m*N*) in 1 and 2 respectively

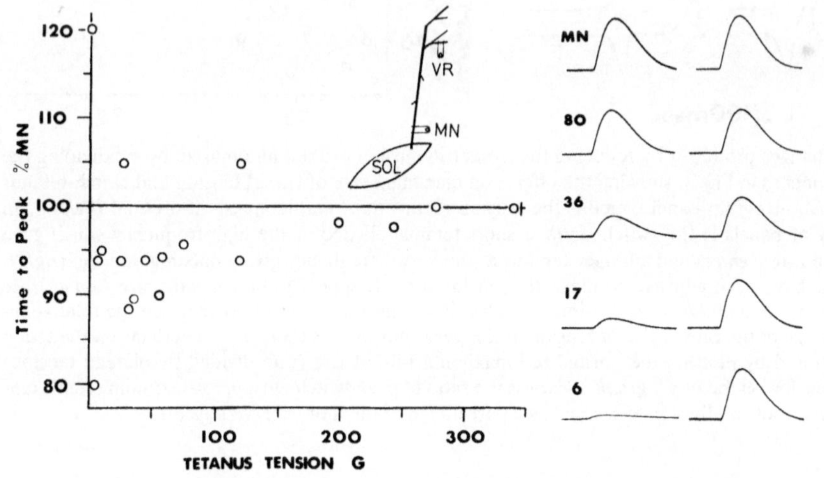

Fig. 3. Effects of decreasing relative compliance by reducing the twitch tension by stimulating ventral root divisions (see diagram). Each pair of myograms shows on the *left* a twitch elicited from a ventral root subdivision recorded at the same gain as the twitch elicited from the motor nerve *(MN)*. The number gives the peak tension as a percentage of MN tension. The myograms on the *right* are recorded at higher gains to show changes in shape. The graph shows how time to peak falls as the twitches are made smaller and produce less extension of the common tendon. Note from the myograms that time to half relaxation increases as time to peak decreases

ing twitches of a muscle linked to the tension transducer by a stiff rod and then replacing the rod with a helical spring (experiments done with C. Rosendorff at King's College, London).It can be seen that when shortening is allowed, serious distortion occurs – twitch tension is reduced with a prolongation of the contraction phase and a shortening of relaxation.

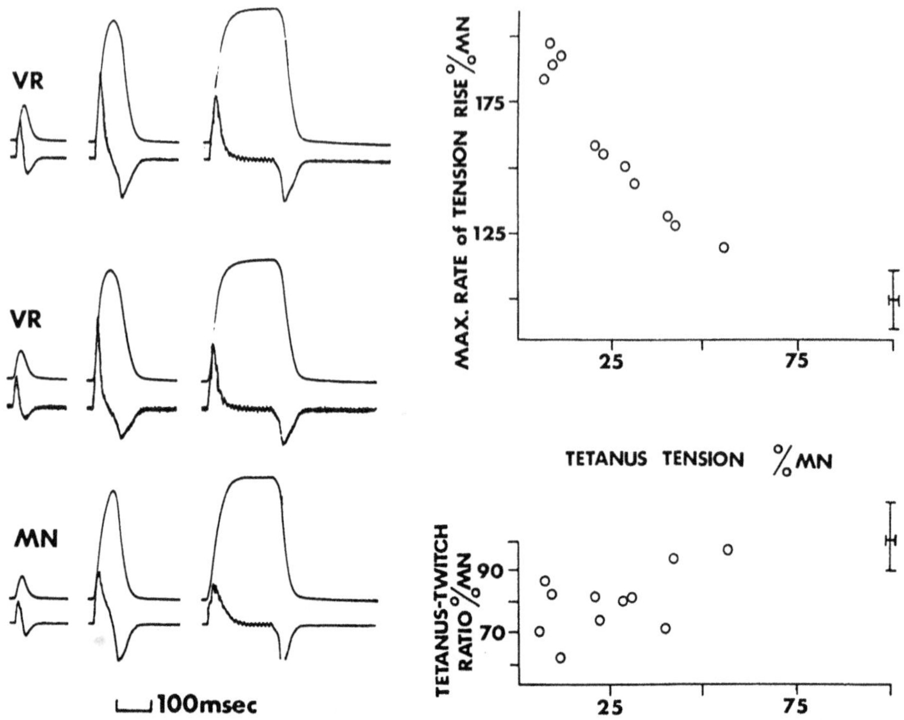

Fig. 4. Changes produced by reducing the isometric tension evoked in a muscle by subdividing the ventral roots as in Fig. 3, showing the effects on maximum rate of rise of tension and twitch-tetanus ratio. Each myogram panel contains the tension record *(top)* and its quasi-differential *(below)*. In each row of panels is the twitch *(left)*, a short tetanus elicited at the high frequency which gave maximum rate *(centre)* and a longer tetanus at the lowest frequency giving maximal tension *(right)*. The gains have been adjusted to make the tension records appear to be the same size *(upper trace* about 5 times and *middle trace* 10 times gain for *MN* – motor nerve) in order to see the relative increase in size of the rate of rise of tension as the peak tension was reduced. The effects on the tetani are illustrated by plotting the normalized maximum rate of rise (rate divided by plateau tension) against tension on the *upper graph*. *Below* is the ratio of peak twitch tension to maximum tetanic tension for the root subdivision expressed as a percentage of the motor nerve tension

The opposite effect may be observed by reducing the extension in a compliant connector or long tendon by comparing a maximal contraction with a submaximal one. In experiments by Lewis and Rosendorff (1964) submaximal contractions were produced by splitting ventral roots into successively smaller fractions (which still contained a sufficient number of motor units to reduce bias due to selection). It can be seen in Fig. 3 that the twitch time to peak was shorter and time to half relaxation longer as the tension and degree of shortening were reduced – the opposite of the effect of increased compliance. Figure 3 shows that the effect on time to peak reached about 10%. Much larger effects (Fig. 4) were found on the maximum rate of rise of tension and on twitch: tetanus ratio. In these experiments the linkage allowed less than 1 mm of shortening in a maximal tetanus in muscles which were more than 60 mm long.

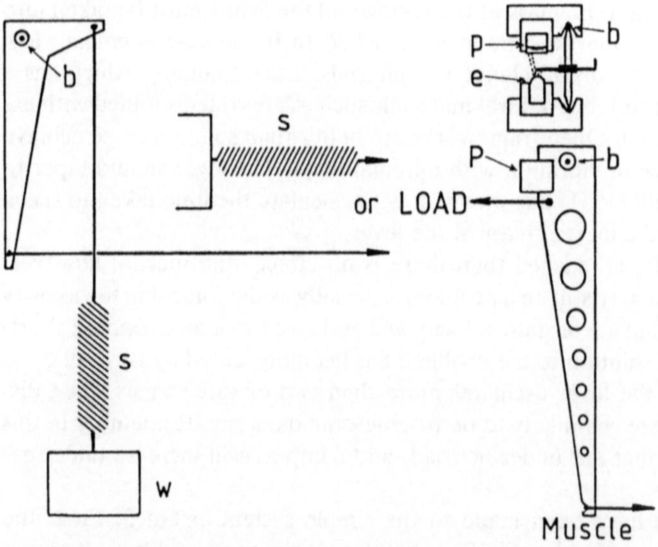

Fig. 5. Simple apparatus for isotonic shortening. The light weight lever is mounted on low friction bearings *(b)* and its movement measured with position detector *(P)*. A convenient detector is shown and consists of a light-emitting diode *(e)* and a photocell *(p)* with a square area (side 1mm) and integral amplifier (R. S. Ltd., 308-067). The load is applied near the axis of rotation and may consist of a long light spring held in tension *(above)* or *(below)* by a weight connected via a spring and a secondary lever which increases the lever ratio and changes the direction of the force. Front and back stops are adjustable for different muscles

Isotonic Recording

The relationship between load or force on the muscle and the resulting constant velocity of shortening after stimulation is shown in Fig. 6. Traditionally isotonic recording is made by attaching the muscle to one end of a light-weight lever which rotates through an axis at the opposite end on low friction bearings. The load is applied nearer to the axis of movement (Fig. 5) in order to reduce inertial effects. Two stops are usually provided, one to prevent the load acting on the muscle before it is stimulated, the other to prevent overshortening. Movement of the lever must be monitored by a device which does not appreciably increase the mass of the lever or damp its movement. A photo cell or a very light induction transducer or similar device can be used. Alternatively, a rotation transducer may be used as the axle for the lever, many low inertia low friction devices are available for servo-control systems.

The load may be a long helical spring stretched to produce the required tension. The length is necessary because its extension must be a small proportion of its length otherwise tension in the spring will rise. Attaching near the axis also helps reduce such an error. If the direction of the load is vertical it is convenient to stretch the spring with a weight, and this can often be achieved with a dual lever system (Fig. 5) which also minimizes effects of inertia. If the lever ratio is R the mass employed will have to be increased by R, but the acceleration of the mass will be reduced by R^2 so the overall inertial load will change by R/R^2, i.e. it is reduced by the lever ratio. It should be remembered that the mass of the spring and the levers must be taken into account when calculating inertia. The lever attached to the muscle is crucial; low mass may be achieved by careful choice of materials. I use titanium, which has a good density: stiffness ratio, but natural materials such as grass stems joined with expoxy resin have been used. Open frameworks are better than solid levers to achieve good stiff structures free of vibration with minimal mass. The lever should taper to reduce inertial mass. Hill (1951) has shown how to calculate the time taken to reach constant velocity from the inertial mass of the lever.

If a constant velocity is reached then there is no effect from inertia; however, damping in the bearings may still be a problem especially as the force due to viscosity or friction will be constant at constant velocity and add an extra load to oppose shortening of the muscle. A solution to the problem has been presented by Birdsall et al. (1977), but, simply, if the lever oscillates more than two or three times when displaced and released there is unlikely to be troublesome damping. Remember in this test that the lever bearings are under no load, and damping will increase under experimental conditions.

Two improvements have been made to the simple system of Fig. 5. First, the lever may be actively restrained until after stimulation has produced full activation of the muscle. This is probably not necessary for all but the most critical recording, since it is shown that full activation of the muscle occurs early after the onset of stimulation (before full isometric tension develops). Moreover, it is difficult to produce a sufficiently rapid release without setting up oscillations. The second possibility is to use a special rotary motor as a mounting for the lever. The current through the motor can be controlled to provide the constant force opposing movement. Further current can be controlled electronically so that the onset of shortening can be timed to occur after the start of stimulation.

The maximum velocity of shortening can be measured by recording isometric tension but arranging that the length of the muscle is suddenly reduced. The reduction should be less than 5% of muscle length and faster than the muscle can shorten. Under these conditions tension falls to zero until the muscle shortens enough to take up the slack. This shortening is at minimum load and therefore at maximum velocity, which may be calculated from the distance moved and the time for redevelopment of tension. The onset of the latter is often difficult to measure, and it may be easier to make the measurements with several steps of length. The method has been described by Hill (1970).

Another alternative is to allow the muscle to shorten at a velocity controlled by a special device; the muscle tension can then be measured. The results obtained match those described above in which load is controlled. This method of measurement has been called isokinetic and has also been described by Hill (1970).

Muscle Stimulation

In isometric recordings, the dynamic properties are most frequently examined in the single twitch and in a fused tetanus. Isotonically the twitch can be recorded but normally only the tetanus is used. In order to understand how such records can be interpreted it is necessary to consider the difference between a twitch and tetanus. The twitch is elicited by a single stimulus from which an action potential propagates all over the muscle surface sarcolemma. Activity also spreads down the transverse (T) tubules towards the centre of the fibre causing the release of ionic calcium. Calcium allows the interaction of the myosin and actin in the thick and thin filaments leading to the development of tension or to shortening of the fibre. Finally calcium is pumped out of the cytosol into the longitudinal elements of the sarcoplasmic reticulum, so that the muscle relaxes. It is thought that in a single twitch in mammalian muscle at body temperature the transient increase in the level of calcium does not reach a level at which the actin-myosin reaction is maximum, perhaps because the T-tubule action potential does not propagate right into the centre of the fibre. In the tetanus, calcium builds up above the saturation level and actin-myosin interaction proceeds at maximum rates. Thus the tension in an isometric tetanus is maximal and only depends in a major way on the length of the muscle. There is an optimal degree of stretch at which there are a maximal number of active sites on the thick and thin filaments in opposition, and force will also be maximal (Gordon et al. 1966). A fall in temperature will produce a small reduction in tension, but a tetanus is relatively insensitive to external factors. Tension will be maximal when the muscle is stimulated with stimuli at an interval which is about 40%–50% of the twitch time to peak (measured from the initial rise in tension to its peak). If the stimulus rate is increased the final tension of the tetanus does not increase, but tension rises more rapidly (Buller and Lewis 1965). Figure 4 illustrates isometric tetani and their differentials from which the maximum rate of rise of tension is measured. The maximal rate of rise of tension is reached at a frequency some five times higher than that necessary to elicit maximal tension (Buller and Lewis 1965). The maximum rate of rise of tension is thought to be determined by the rate of formation of cross-bridges between myosin of the thick and actin of the thin filaments.

Similar considerations apply to isotonic tetani. Stimulation rates about three times those necessary for maximum isometric tetani tension give fastest shortening (i.e. less than that necessary for maximum rate of rise of isometric tension). The velocity of shortening is also dependent on actin-myosin interaction rates, but it is thought that the rate limiting step is different to that involved in the isometric tetanus – the rate of breakage of cross-links is important in muscle shortening. It is not surprising, therefore, that the maximum rate of rise of tetanic isometric tension and the maximum velocity of isotonic shortening vary together among types of muscle and species. At long or short muscle lengths, at which tension is low, the rate of rise of tension and velocity of shortening are both reduced proportionately. Temperature has an effect on both rates and velocity and the Q_{10} is large – over two (Ranatunga 1983). Few other factors affect these variables, in contrast to the changes listed below for the twitch. Differential changes, however, have been observed under abnormal conditions (e.g. after denervation, Kean et al. 1974).

Thus, tetani, whether isometric or isotonic, depend largely on the biochemical properties of the myofibrillar contractile proteins. Muscle activation is maximal (at least after the first few milliseconds) and does not contribute to the pattern of contraction. In the twitch, however, calcium release is transient (Eusebi et al. 1980) and probably submaximal. The time course and amplitude of the twitch depends, therefore, on the rates of release and reuptake of calcium by the sarcoplasmic reticulum as well as on the properties of the contractile proteins. The following description will be of isometric twitches but would apply to isotonic ones if they were recorded. The form of the twitch can be affected by the number of external factors, some of which are described below. At short lengths the tension will be smaller and the time course briefer; at long lengths contraction and relaxation are longer. A fall of temperature slows twitches, again with a high Q_{10}; its effect on peak tension depends on the type of the muscle, increasing tension in fast muscle and decreasing it in slow-twitch muscle. A preceding tetanus potentiates a fast muscle twitch with little change in the time course; slow muscle twitch tension is depressed whilst time to peak and half relaxation both fall (in proportion to the change in tension). The effects of adrenaline (β action) resemble those of a preceding tetanus in some way. Slow muscle is some five times more sensitive and the twitch times to peak and half are reduced with only a slight fall in tension. The fast muscle twitch is potentiated by adrenaline (at levels above those found naturally), with prolongation of the contraction and relaxation phases. It can be seen, therefore, that recording conditions have a marked effect on the twitch, although differences between fast and slow muscle always remain distinct.

Despite these multiple factors there is normally a close relationship between the parameters of the twitch and tetanus. Thus, a fast muscle has a brief twitch, rapid shortening under isotonic conditions and a high rate of rise of tension in a tetanic tension. Close (1972) has quantitated the relationships between these first two variables. He has plotted the maximum velocity of isotonic tetanic shortening against the reciprocal of the isometric twitch time to peak (taking the reciprocal converts a time to a type of rate). To achieve a wide range of variables Close took data from a number of species ranging in speed of muscle contraction from mouse to man and at several different temperatures (allowing nonmammalian species to be compared). A continuous, linear relationship over two decades was observed. This general relationship indicates that in normal muscles the processes controlling the release and reuptake of calcium following a single stimulus are closely matched to the rate of interaction of the contractile proteins. This arrangement has the clear advantage that it will give optimal muscle performance, but it should be realised that it involves very close matching of a number of genetic systems which must be necessary to determine so many aspects of muscle contraction. Undoubtedly the trophic effect of a nerve (Buller et al. 1960a), which determines many aspects of muscle biochemistry, serves to coordinate the activation and contractile processes. It should be noted, however, that there are also genetic factors (Buller et al. 1960b) which are important in determining twitch (Lewis 1973) and shortening (El-Mubarak and Ranatunga 1985) properties, so the correlation between shortening velocity and twitch time course must also involve coordination of gene expression.

Breakdown of the Relationship Between Twitch Time to Peak and Isotonic Shortening Velocity

Close, who drew attention to the reciprocal relation between isometric twitch time to peak and isotonic shortening velocity which is seen when examining a wide range of muscles, also demonstrated that the relationship did not hold up when looked at in detail in particular muscles. Close and Luff (1974) compared the extensor digitorum longus (EDL, a fast muscle) from the rat hind limb with the inferior rectus muscle of the eye. It had been known for some time (Cooper and Eccles 1930) that the isometric twitch contraction of the extrinsic eye muscles have a time course which is less than half that of limb fast muscles. Close and Luff confirmed the difference in the rat but found that the differences between isometric shortening velocities were very small: the inferior rectus shortened only 10% faster than EDL. They suggested that the eye muscle twitch was fast because activation was very brief, disproportionately so in relation to the intrinsic speed of interaction of actin and myosin. As well as causing the twitch to be short, the brief calcium transient did not allow twitch tension to develop fully. The ratio of twitch to tetanic tension is about 0.15 in EDL and other fast twitch muscles, but in inferior rectus it was as low as 0.05.

More recently Wilson and Woledge (1985) have re-examined this problem in single fibres dissected from frog tibialis anterior. Amphibian muscle contains some five fibre types with a wide range of contraction speeds. Wilson and Woledge found a correlation between maximum velocity of shortening and maximum rate of rise of isometric twitch tension. Neither variable was correlated with twitch time to peak, again indicating a dissociation between activation and the properties of the contractile proteins.

Dissociation, but in the opposite direction, is seen in the response of rat EDL to denervation. Within a few days of axotomy the twitch times to peak and half relaxation increase by more than 50% (e.g. Finol et al. 1981). This is not matched by changes in shortening velocity, which falls by only 10% (Baker and Lewis 1982). As might be expected from the earlier arguments, there is a threefold increase in the twitch: tetanus ratio. Qualitatively similar changes were observed in rat soleus (slow twitch muscle), although qualitatively there was a smaller mismatch between isometric twitch prolongation and shortening velocity reduction.

The change in the twitch following denervation may be described as a prolongation increase in the active state (e.g. Hill 1970). Finol et al. (1981) suggested that the active state might be increased by a larger and longer release of calcium into the cytosol by the prolongation of the muscle fibre action potential which is characteristic of denervation. More recently Dulhunty and Gate (1985) have proposed an alternative (or additional) mechanism – an increase in excitation-contraction coupling. The observed that denervated muscle produced a larger tension in response to membrane depolarisation. This could be due to, for example, a greater release of calcium to a given level of depolarisation or to greater sensitivity to calcium of the formation of cross bridges between thick and thin filaments.

Chronic Stimulation of Denervated Muscle

In 1974 Lømo et al. observed the effects on denervated rat soleus of long-term stimulation with intermittant short bursts of stimuli at 100 Hz. They found that the twitch became much briefer, approximating to that of fast muscle. This was a very important observation because it indicated that the activity of muscle alone could produce

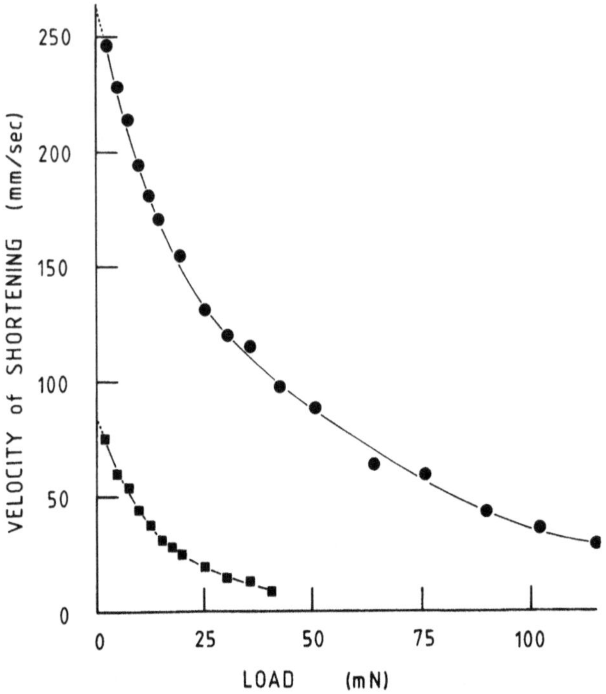

Fig. 6. Isotonic velocities plotted against load on the muscle. The *squares* are of rat soleus denervated for 29 days. The *circles* are from the contralateral soleus also denervated but stimulated by 1-s bursts of pulses every 90 s for 10 h a day

changes in the muscle properties – the postulated chemical neurotrophic factor proposed by Buller et al. (1960b) could not be involved in denervated muscle. It remained possible, however, that the observed change could be due to changes in activation alone. That is to say, the stimulation might only be modifying one group of muscle properties, and the difference between stimulated denervated muscle and denervated muscle might be equivalent to the difference between the inferior rectus and EDL discussed above.

It was important, therefore, to examine the isotonic shortening velocity directly. We used methods of stimulation similar to those of Lømo et al. (1974) for chronic stimulation and examined isotonic shortening velocities of the chronically stimulated muscles (Al-Amood and Lewis 1983). A typical experiment is illustrated in Fig. 6, in which a chronically stimulated denervated rat soleus is compared with the contralateral muscle denervated at the same time. Two effects can be seen. First the stimulated muscle is able to shorten against larger loads, corresponding to the increased isometric tetanic tension. Secondly there is a marked increase in the maximum velocity of shortening in the stimulated muscle not only above that of denervated soleus (which has a lower than normal velocity) but also faster than normal soleus. The highest velocities were about 300 mm/s which are close to those of soleus muscle cross-reinnervated by EDL nerve and subsequently denervated (298 mm/s, SD = 33 mm/s, n = 8: Baker and Lewis 1982). We conclude, therefore, that the stimulation pattern used by Lømo and Westgaard transforms the contractile proteins of slow muscle to an extent similar to that produced by fast nerve innervation, and that there is no dissociation of the two aspects of muscle contractile properties.

We have, however, found some differences from the results of Lømo et al. The change in twitch time to peak was from 32 ms in control soleus to about 20 ms in our stimulated denervated muscles, which was slower than the twitches recorded by Lømo et al. (13 ms). Another difference was that over the 2–3 month period used for stimulation we found that there was a progressive reduction in the twitch time to peak of unstimulated denervated muscles. Denervation for 7–20 days causes the time to peak to increase to 45 ms (Finol et al. 1981; Baker and Lewis 1982). After several months the time to peak fell by 28 ms to 27 ms. This fall is some 70% of that in the stimulated denervated muscle (which fell by 25 ms to 20 ms). A late speeding up of denervated rat soleus had been described by Gutmann et al. (1972) who also showed that the transformation was accompanied by an increase in ATPase activity (correlated with shortening velocity). We have found some increase in the shortening velocity in long-term denervated muscles compared with early denervations, but these experiments are difficult because the tetanic tension falls some 50-fold whereas the passive tension due to connective tissue does not fall and may even rise. As a result, when small loads are used to examine the highest velocities of shortening, the load will be less than the passive tension and the muscle will shorten due to the elasticity. If passive shortening is more than 1 mm, the thick and thin filaments will be moved out of the region of maximum interaction and the velocity of shortening

Table 1. Effects of stimulation on denervated rat soleus muscle. In the muscles summarized in *rows 1–11* bursts of pulses lasting 1 s at the frequency given in column 1 were repeated at the intervals of column 2. The duration of stimulation is shown in column 3. All muscles stimulated at 100 Hz were restricted to about 10 h but the rest were for 24 h a day. *Row 12* describes muscles stimulated continuously. *Rows 13 and 14* are denervated muscles left unstimulated. *Row 15* is data for normal muscles from rats of similar age and weight (Baker and Lewis 1982)

Frequency (Hz)	Interval (s)	Duration (days)	Tetanic tension (m*N*)		
			Mean	*n*	SEM
100	10	49	336	3	41
100	30	62	214	5	45
100	60	46	237	3	83
100	90	50	302	5	85
60	90	38	384	5	112
40	60	36	523	3	63
40	90	42	673	3	157
40	300	55	465	3	34
40	600	56	229	2	217
20	90	56	337	3	116
10	90	28	132	3	21
10	Continuous	36	220	3	33
0	–	20	241	8	13
0	–	47	46	7	9
0	(Control)	–	2090	6	250

will be reduced. Under these conditions the force-velocity curves fall off again at low loads. When active tension falls too much, excessive extrapolation of the force-velocity curve would have to be done with a very uncertain estimate of maximum velocity. The possibility must remain that stimulation is simply exaggerating a spontaneous transformation of denervated muscle, perhaps by reducing atrophy differentially.

Our experiments have also examined effects of changing the frequency used in chronic stimulation (Al-Amood et al. 1985). In the experiments reported above by Lømo et al. and by ourselves short bursts of stimuli were given using frequencies of 100 Hz. The interval between the bursts could be from 10 s up to 2 h (Lømo et al. 1980). We have used bursts at intervals ranging from 10 to 600 s with frequencies of 100, 60, 40, 20 and 10 Hz, and found that the greatest effect on tension and twitch time to peak was produced by 40–60 Hz, although all frequencies produced the effect and there were no statistically significant differences. We conclude from these experiments that high-frequency stimulation is not necessary, but that intermittancy may be the important factor. We confirmed the observation of Lømo et al. that continuous stimulation at 10 Hz maintains a slow contraction in denervation soleus.

The effects of these stimulation regimes on muscle force are shown in Table 1. Because the experiments were designed for different purposes, the regimes varied in more than one parameter. It is clear, however, that all patterns maintained muscle tension at a level equivalent to less than 20 days denervation for periods of at least 60 days. There was some variation in the tension of the stimulated denervated muscles, but none of the variation appeared to be related to stimulation parameters except, perhaps, that continuous stimulation was less effective in maintaining muscle force than intermittant stimulation. It should be noted that the tensions of the stimulated muscles were never more than a quarter of those of muscles from normal animals. Caution is recommended when extrapolating these data to fast twitch muscles, which are known to atrophy more slowly following denervation.

One final stimulation pattern was tested because we thought that the long high-frequency bursts used by us and Lømo were unlikely to occur naturally. It has been observed, however, that there is often a brief high-frequency burst at the beginning of muscle contraction, often just a doublet of spikes. We therefore tried stimulating with a pair of pulses spaced at 5 ms and repeated every 60 s. The effects were inconsistent but in two out of four experiments the twitch became as fast as in muscles stimulated by long bursts.

In conclusion, we have shown that muscles that are chronically stimulated show a speeding up. Changes are seen both in the isometric twitch and the isotonic tetanus suggesting that both the activation processes and the contractile proteins are modified in parallel. The effects of this type of chronic stimulation are, therefore, similar to those produced by reinnervation by a nerve from a fast-twitch muscle. Some uncertainty must remain about the interpretation since similar but smaller effects are seen if denervated muscles are left unstimulated for the same length of time.

References

Al-Amood WS, Lewis DM (1983) Isotonic responses of chronically stimulated denervated rat soleus muscle. J Physiol (Lond) 338: 15P

Al-Amood WS, Lewis DM, Rowlerson A (1985) The effects of chronic stimulation at low rates on denervated rat soleus muscle. J Physiol (Lond) 361:36P

Baker AJ, Lewis DM (1982) The effects of denervation on isotonic shortening velocity of rat fast and slow muscle. J Physiol (Lond) 345:56P

Birdsall DL, Hodgson JA, Lewis DM (1977) Evaluation of an isotonic apparatus for muscle recording. J Physiol (Lond) 265:10–11P

Brooks D (1984) Improved reliability of tendon force transducers. Biological Engineering Scoiety

Buller AJ, Lewis DM (1963) Factors affecting the differentiation of mammalian fast and slow muscle fibres. In: Gutmann E, Hnik P (eds) Proceedings of symposium on the effect of use and disuse on neuromusclular functions. Czechoslovak Acadamy of Science, Prague, pp 149–160

Buller AJ, Lewis DM (1965) The rate of tension development in isometric tetanic contractions of mammalian fast and slow skeletal muscle. J Physiol (Lond) 176:337–354

Buller AJ, Eccles JC, Eccles RM (1960a) Differentiation of fast and slow muscles in the cat hind limb. J Physiol (Lond) 150:399–416

Buller AJ, Eccles JC, Eccles RM (1960b) Interaction between motoneurones and muscles in respect of the characteristic speed of their responses. J Physiol (Lond) 150:417–439

Close R (1965) The relation between intrinsic speed of shortening and duration of the active state in muscle. J Physiol (Lond) 180:542–559

Close RI (1972) Dynamic properties of mammalian skeletal muscles. Physiol Rev 52:129–197

Close R, Luff AR (1974) Dynamic properties of inferior rectus muscle of the rat. J Physiol (Lond) 236:259–270

Cooper S. Eccles JC (1930) The isometric responses of mammalian muscles. J Physiol (Lond) 69:377–385

Dulhunty AF, Gage PW (1985) Excitation-contraction coupling and charge movement in denervated rat extensor digitorum longus and soleus muscles. J Physiol (Lond) 358:75–89

Elmurbarak MH, Ranatunga KW (1985) The effects of denervation on post-natal changes in the isotonic shortening velocity of rat fast and slow-twitch muscles. J Physiol (Lond) 364:40P

Eusebi F, Miledi R, Takahashi T (1980) Calcium transients in mammalian muscle. Nature 284:560–561

Finol HJ, Lewis DM, Owens R (1981) The effects of denervation on contractile properties of rat skeletal muscle. J Physiol (Lond) 319:81–92

Gordon AM, Huxley AF, Julian FJ (1966) The variation in isometric tension with sarcomere length in vertebrate muscle fibres. J Physiol (Lond) 184:170–173

Gutmann E, Melinchna J, Syrovy I (1972) Contraction properties and ATPase activity in fast and slow muscle of the rat during denervation. Exp Neurol 36:488–497

Hill AV (1951) The transition from rest to full activity in muscle. Proc R Soc Lond [Biol] 138:329–345

Hill AV (1970) First and last experiments in muscle mechanics. Cambridge University Press, Cambridge

Hodgson JA (1982) Methods of recording muscle activity in conscious cats to assess involvement in movement. J Physiol (Lond) 327:13P

Kean CJS, Lewis DM, McGarrick JD (1974) Dynamic properties of denervated fast and slow twitch muscle of the cat. J Physiol (Lond) 237:103–113

Lewis DM (1973) Effect of denervation on the differentiation of twitch muscles of the kitten hind limb. Nature 241:285–286

Lewis DM, Rosendorff C (1964) The contraction times of submaximal twitches of mammalian fast and slow skeletal muscles. J Physiol (Lond) 177:55–56P

Lømo T, Westgaard RH, Dahl HA (1974) Contractile properties of muscle: control by pattern of muscle activity in the rat. Proc R Soc Lond [Biol] 187:99–103

Lømo T, Westgaard RH, Engebretsen L (1980) Different stimulation patterns affect contractile properties of denervated rat soleus muscle. In: Pette D (ed) Plasticity of muscle. deGruyter, Berlin, pp 297–309

Ranatunga KW (1983) Influence of temperature on the shortening velocity of rat skeletal muscle. J Physiol (Lond) 341:40–41P

Wilson MGA, Woledge RC (1985) Lack of correlation between twitch contraction time and velocity of unloaded shortening in fibres of frog anterior tibialis muscle. J Physiol (Lond) 358:81P

Effect of Electrical Stimulation on Denervated Muscle

W. A. Nix[1]

Introduction

The possibilities of noninvasive treatment in peripheral nerve injuries are limited. Although it is well known that the severance of a nerve results in paralysis of the dependent tissue, the methods of treating a denervated muscle are still controversial. The most obvious result of denervation is muscle atrophy and paralysis. In 1841 Reid forced the denervated muscle to contract by electrical stimulation to replace the loss of activity and observed that this treatment retarded atrophy. Since then, there has been continuing interest in preventing muscle atrophy with electrotherapy. Peripheral nerve injuries in the two world wars were, for instance, extensively treated with electrical stimulation. However, the usefulness of this therapeutic regime has been doubtful since reports of the success of the treatment are far from uniform. To date there have been no rigorous studies to evaluate the beneficial effect of this procedure in patients. Along with the clinical trials animal experiments have been conducted, yet many of these are impossible to compare, because the conditions of the experiments, such as stimuli parameters, duration of treatment, and conditions under which the muscle contracted, were too different. The best study conducted to date was that of Gutmann and Guttmann in 1944. They proved morphologically an atrophy-retarding effect of electrical stimulation in rabbit extensor digitorum longus (EDL). The results were dependent on controlled experimental conditions; treatment had to be applied each day for at least 20 min and the elicited muscle contraction had to be vigorous.

Little was known at that time about the influence the nerve exerts upon muscle. In 1960 Buller et al. demonstrated that cross-reinnervation of a fast or a slow muscle with a nerve normally supplying a slow or a fast muscle, respectively, induced a change in contractile characteristics. A trophic factor was presumed to be the main mediator of these changes. Salmons and Vrbová showed in 1969 that activity also plays a major role. The transformation of innervated fast rabbit EDL into a slow twitch muscle was achieved by superimposing, via implanted electrodes, a frequency pattern which is normally delivered to a slow-twitch muscle by its own motoneuron. Further experiments showed that changes induced by activity included transformation of biochemical and structural characteristics (Pette et al. 1976) The influence of this type of stimulation on denervated rabbit EDL has not yet been studied.

In this study the effects of either long-term or short-term low-frequency stimulation on contractile and morphological properties of the denervated fast-twitch EDL were examined.

1 Department of Neurology, University Clinics, Johannes-Gutenberg University, Mainz, West Germany

Electrical Stimulation and Neuromuscular Disorders
Ed. by W. A. Nix and G. Vrbová

Methods

Experiments were performed on rabbits of either sex of about 2.5–3 kg body weight. The animals were divided into three groups, a denervated control ($n = 26$), a denervated and 1 Hz stimulated ($n = 12$) and a denervated and 8 Hz stimulated group ($n = 11$). In all groups the EDL muscle of one leg was denervated; the experimental sides (left or right) were chosen alternately to exclude possible side-dependent differences in the muscle. Using pentobarbital as an anaesthetic (30 mg/kg) and with sterile precautions the peroneal nerve was exposed in the thigh and a 2–3-cm-long piece excised. The proximal and distal stumps were folded and tied with a thread. These nerve stumps were then sewn into the surrounding musculature to prevent reinnervation. In all animals two electrodes were implanted, one at the proximal end of the muscle between the EDL muscle and the tibia, the other over the distal third of the EDL. The fascia covering the EDL and tibialis anterior muscle was left intact while securing the electrodes onto it. Surgical trauma to the denervated muscle was thus minimized. The wire electrodes were connected to an insulated lead, led under the skin and externalised at the back of the animal, where they were attachted to a plug that the animal carried on a plastic saddle.

The stimulating electrodes were prepared from multistranded flexible steel wire (Ethicon 619p, Norderstedt). An elliptic loop with the long diameter of 1.5 cm was formed. The rest of the wire was insulated by threading the blank wires into silicon tubing (Silastic, Dow Corning, Düsseldorf).

The animals in the stimulated groups were connected to a stimulator (Grass Medical Instruments S88, Quincy, Mass.) 2 days after the operation and were stimulated for 4 weeks. The polarity was reversed after each stimulus to minimize possible damage caused by polarisation of the tissue.

In the 8-Hz group, stimuli of 1-ms pulse width with a frequency of 8 Hz were used. The stimulus strength was adjusted so that vigorous muscle contractions were obtained with visible movements of the paw. Fifteen minutes of continuous stimulation were alternated with a 15-min rest, averaging the time of effective stimulation to 12 h per day.

In the 1-Hz group, the denervated muscle was stimulated daily with 1 Hz for 20 min. Square-wave pulses with a 7-ms pulse width were used. In this group, care was taken to achieve isometric muscle contraction. This could only be done by placing the hindlimb in a plaster cast with the knee flexed and the foot extended. Vigorous contractions were obtained by adjusting the stimulating current without applying painful stimuli. Upon palpation of the muscle the vigorous contractions could be felt.

Physiological Recordings

Thirty days after denervation and after 28 days of stimulation the animals were anaesthetized intravenously with Nembutal (30 mg/kg) and the final experiments were performed. The legs were rigidly fixed with a drill through the proximal and distal tibia and fastened to a steel plate. The distal tendon of the EDL was freed and attached to a strain gauge. Care was taken to maintain the muscle temperature at

37°C throughout the experiment using a thermoprobe in the muscle connected to a heating lamp. To avoid drying of the muscle and surrounding tissues, a skin pouch was formed and filled with paraffin oil. By means of a micromanipulator, the length of the muscle was adjusted to produce the maximal tension on stimulation. The following parameters were measured: mechanical latency, contraction time, ½ relaxation time, twitch and tetanic force. Tetanic tension was obtained by stimulating the muscle at 100 Hz for 350 ms. The susceptibility to fatigue was measured as described by Burke et al. (1971). The stimulus parameters were modified so that the muscles were stimulated each second at 40 Hz for 300 ms. The fatigue index was expressed as a percentage of the tension after 3 min when initial tension was taken to be 100%. In the final experiment the implanted electrodes were used for the stimulation of the denervated muscles. Supramaximal square-wave pulses with a width of 1 ms were used.

Histological Examination

Both control and stimulated muscles were excised and weighed. A section from the middle portion of the muscle was prepared and frozen in liquid nitrogen. In denervated muscles that were chronically stimulated larger muscle fibres were observed under the electrodes. To avoid artifacts, the middle part of the muscle, which was not in close contact with the electrodes, was studied. Cryostat sections of denervated and control muscles (thickness: 6 μm) were put on the same slide to process under identical conditions for succinic dehydrogenase, van Gieson and haematoxylin-eosin (Dubowitz and Brooke 1973). For measurements of fibre diameter, microphotographs were taken and enlarged (260 ×). The lesser diameter of the muscle fibre was measured according to Dubowitz and Brooke (1973) on paper prints using a digitising tablet (Cardio 80, Kontron) connected to a microprocessor. The program for these measurments was marketed by Kontron. No correction was made for obliquity of section or irregularities in muscle fibres.

Results

Mechanical Latency

Mechanical latency is the time that elapses between the stimulus and the onset of the twitch. As can be seen in Table 1, denervation prolongs the period from 4.7 to 5.2 ms. Different stimulation regimes had no effect on this parameter and did not influence the denervation-induced prolongation of the mechanical latency.

Contraction and Half Relaxation Times

Innervated EDL muscle had a fast contraction time of 22.5 ± 2.0 ms as well as a fast ½ relaxation time of 15.4 ± 3.9 ms (Table 1). Four weeks after denervation these

Table 1. Parameters for normal and denervated muscle for controls and for denervated muscle stimulated with short-term 1-Hz or long-term 8-Hz regimens

Different parameters	For	Control group			1-Hz group				8-Hz stimulated group			
		n	$\bar{x}$	s	n	$\bar{x}$	s	P	n	$\bar{x}$	s	P
Mechanical latency (ms)	N	26	4.7	0.5								
	D	26	5.2	0.6	10	6.1	0.5	0.09	10	5.3	0.4	0.357
Contraction time (ms)	N	26	22.5	2.0								
	D	26	33.6	2.6	10	31.1	1.5	$0.44 \cdot 10^{-2}$	11	35.3	3.7	0.04
Twitch : tetanus	N	25	0.33	0.1								
	D	25	0.61	0.13	9	0.47	0.04	0.01	10	0.60	0.15	0.43
Fatigue index	N	20	0.35	0.08								
	D	20	0.62	0.11	12	0.50	0.1	0.006	10	0.47	0.12	0.003
Diameter (μm)	N	9	50.4	7.35								
	D	9	34.7	8.3	10	42.0	6.4	0.02	10	36.1	7.1	0.36
Area (μm^2)	N	9	3699.5	1102.2								
	D	9	1866.1	810.2	10	2703.6	595.3	0.009	10	1845.8	714.6	0.48

Values are given as means *($\bar{x}$)* for number of animals *(n)* with standard deviation *(s)*. All muscles that were stimulated for 28 days had been denervated for 30 days. The muscle fatigue was calculated as the ratio of the tetanic force after 3 min of intermittent stimulation to the force before minus 1. This index multiplied by 100 represents the difference in percentage of denervated muscle as opposed to normal muscle. Corresponding values for the denervated and denervated stimulated muscles were compared for statistical analysis. Significance *(P)* was assessed on the unpaired data using Student's *t*-test

parameters were prolonged to 33.6 ± 2.6 ms and 29.9 ± 5.9 ms, respectively. Isotonic long-term 8-Hz stimulation made the denervated muscle slower contracting. Short-term isometric 1-Hz stimulation had a different effect; both muscle contraction and ½ relaxation time were faster than in denervated muscle. Compared to denervated only muscle, 1-Hz stimulation maintained a faster speed of contraction whereas 8-Hz stimulation led to a further decrease.

Twitch: Tetanus Ratio

The twitch: tetanus ratio was calculated by dividing the twitch tension by the tetanic tension minus one. Multiplied by one hundred it gives an estimate in percent of the difference between the normal muscle and the denervated or stimulated muscle, respectively. This ratio may be indicative of the duration of the so-called active state of the muscle while contracting. The 8-Hz stimulated denervated muscle showed a value of 0.6 ± 0.15 which does not differ from only denervated muscle. A better performance was seen in the 1-Hz denervated stimulated muscle. This muscle can be ranked between a normal and a denervated one with a ratio of 0.47 ± 0.04.

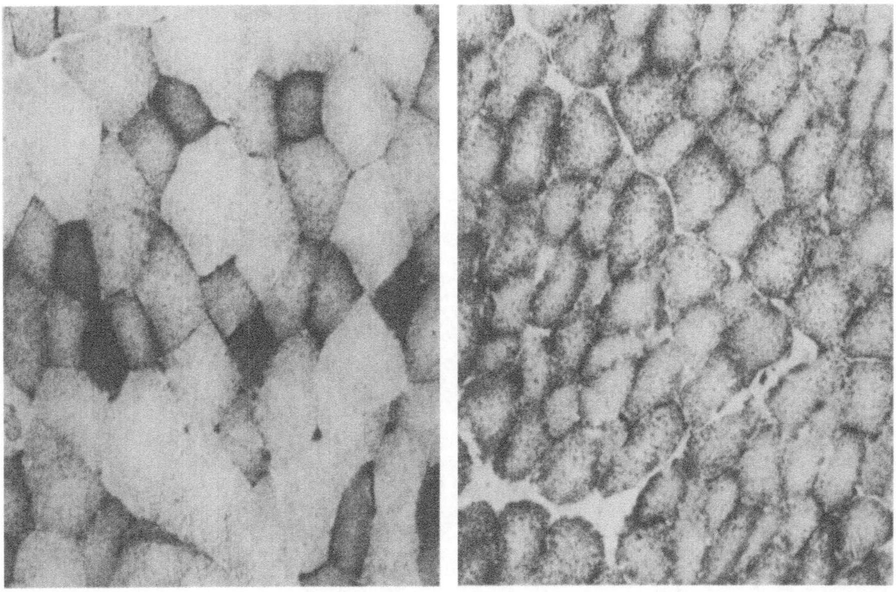

Fig. 1. Histological picture of the EDL of an animal denervated and stimulated with 8 Hz. *Left,* normal innervated side; *right,* denervated stimulated muscle. Both muscles were stained on the same slide under identical conditions for succinic dehydrogenase (× 140). In the normal muscle the staining shows a mosaic-like pattern, whereas the denervated stimulated muscle is intenser and more homogeneous with an subsarcolemmal increase. For only denervated muscles a more homogeneous, but less intense, staining is reported (Nachmias and Padykula 1958). (By courtesy of Prof. Schröder, Dept. of Neuropathology, Aachen)

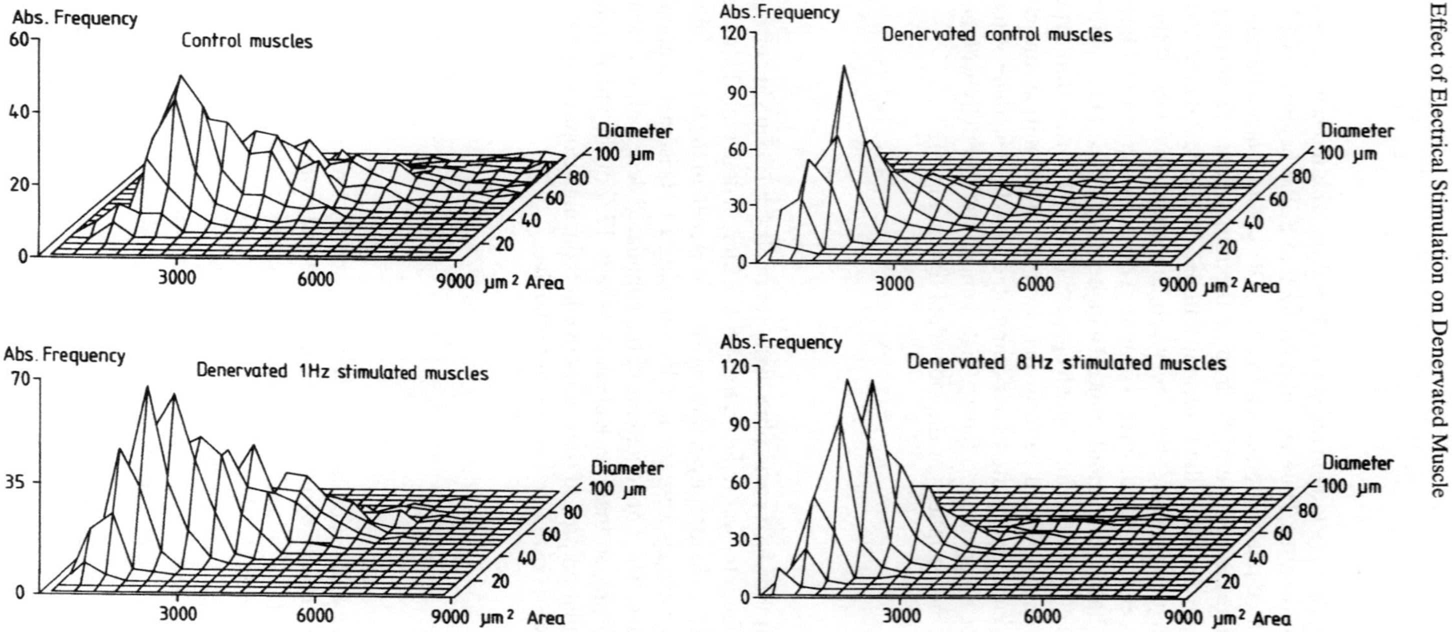

Fig. 2. Correlations of the morphologically evaluated data for the mean fibre diameter and cross-section fibre area according to their absolute frequency. *Upper left,* normal, *upper right,* denervated muscle: a shift to smaller values can be seen. *Lower left,* denervated 1-Hz stimulated muscle *lower right,* denervated 8-Hz stimulated muscles. The 1-Hz stimulated muscles have a similar scatter of values to the control muscles, but tend to be smaller. Denervated control and denervated 8-Hz stimulated muscles have the same distribution of fibre diameters, indicating no effect of electrical stimulation

Fatigue Index

In Table 1 the normal muscle has a fatigue index of 0.35 ± 0.08. This index was calculated by dividing the tension after 3 min stimulation by that at the beginning of it. The tension of the innervated muscle decreased by 35%. Denervation made the muscle fatigue faster, the decrease being a 62% drop of the initial force. Denervated muscle is, therefore, more fatigable than normal muscle. Stimulated denervated muscles become more fatigue-resistant than denervated only ones. No further differences could be seen between the two stimulated groups. This demonstrates that both forms of activity patterns had an effect and induced a higher fatigue resistance. After staining for the oxydative enzyme succinic dehydrogenase (SDH) a muscle fibre type differentiation seen as a chequerboard pattern was observed in the normal muscle but not in the denervated and denervated 1-Hz stimulated muscle. The denervated and 8-Hz stimulated muscle appeared to have a higher mean SDH activity with accumulation of staining in the periphery of the individual fibres (Fig. 1).

Fibre Diameter

Morphological evaluation showed a mean fibre diameter of 50.4 ± 7.35 μm in normal innervated muscle. The diameter was reduced to 34.6 ± 8.2 μm in denervated muscle which is a reduction of 31%. No atrophy-retarding effect was seen in the 8-Hz stimulated group. The atrophic changes were reduced by imposing a 1-Hz isometric stimulation regime on the muscle. The fibre diameter of the stimulated denervated muscle was reduced to 42.0 ± 6.4 μm, so that the decrease was only 17% of the initial fibre diameter. The 1-Hz stimulation proved to be effective in reducing atrophy while the long-term, low-frequency 8-Hz stimulation was not effective.

Discussion

Long-term, low-frequency 8-Hz stimulation as well as a short-term, isometric 1-Hz activity have been shown to be able to influence contractile and morphological parameters in denervated muscle. Following 1-Hz stimulation, the treated muscle performed better than a denervated only muscle. In contrast, 8-Hz stimulation slowed contraction time and increased fatigue resistance but left the rate of atrophy and the twitch : tetanus ratio unaffected. This indicates that different stimulation procedures have their own specific effect on muscle and raise the question of how they are brought about.

Treating denervated muscle while permitting the nerve to regenerate complicates any interpretation of the results because the effects on the muscle alone or via the nerve cannot be differentiated sufficiently (Nix 1982; Girlanda et al. 1982; Cole and Gardiner 1984). The effect of electrical stimulation and denervated muscle cannot be attributed to a possibly altered composition of trophic factors in the nerve, as has been presumed for innervated muscles. If activity of the muscle is involved in the maintenance of contractile and metabolic factors of muscle, then electrically induced contraction should be able to change or maintain the normal muscle composition in the absence of innervation. That this is the case was shown in the study implementing a low-frequency, 8-Hz stimulation.

The fast-twitch, denervated muscle could be changed towards a muscle resembling a slow-twitch muscle. Taking into consideration the 4 weeks of treatment, the changes within the denervated muscle were only slight when compared with the profound alterations in the innervated muscle (Salmons and Vrbová 1969; Pette et al. 1973, 1975, 1976). Stimulation of denervated rabbit EDL muscle for 4 weeks with intermittent 40-Hz bursts and a mean frequency of 4 Hz had no effect at all on the denervated muscle (Nix et al. 1983). A similar stimulation pattern in innervated muscles produced the same degree of slowing of contractile properties as the slow stimulation pattern (Eerbeek et al. 1984).

The activity produced by stimulating the slow-twitch soleus muscle in small animals was shown to prevent loss of oxydative enzymes and the atrophy associated with denervation (Lømo et al. 1974; Nemeth 1982). The changes became more marked when stimulation for longer periods was used. Denervated rat soleus that was stimulated with low frequency for over 2 months maintained the twitch characteristics resembling a normal innervated soleus. High-frequency stimulation, on the other hand, induced fast-twitch contractile parameters in the muscle, and atrophy could be retarded (Lømo et al. 1980). For this study different activity patterns were used on one to three rats. Trains of 100-Hz or 10-Hz bursts with different time intervals resulted in a mean frequency of 1 or 9 Hz. The presence of high-frequency bursts was presumed to regulate the speed of contraction. The amount of activity, rather than the characteristics of frequency, regulated the fatigue behaviour. Hudlická et al. (1980) found this to be so in innervated muscles.

Whether or not long-term stimulation can retard denervation-induced atrophy has not been proven. When innervated EDL muscle is stimulated with a low-frequency pattern, a reduction in fibre diameter and twitch tension can be observed (Salmons and Vrbová 1969; Pette et al. 1975; Eerbeek et al. 1984). In denervated muscle, denervation-induced reduction of fibre cross-sectional area is paralleled by a reduction of fibre diameter as a result of low-frequency stimulation. Therefore, low-frequency stimulation would not be expected to have an atrophy-retarding effect. In denervated, stimulated soleus muscle, atrophy could be retarded with electrical stimulation (Lømo et al. 1980). The difference between these results and those of the present study may be due to the different species of animals used (rat denervated slow soleus muscle versus rabbit denervated fast EDL). The fact that a smaller muscle, such as the rat soleus, lends itself better for stimulation than a larger muscle, like the rabbit EDL, must also be taken into consideration.

The present study also shoes that the amount of activity plays a major role. It influences both fatigue behaviour and contraction time. The enhanced aerobic oxydative capacity of the muscle was expressed by the increase in oxydative enzyme activity. This increase in oxydative enzyme activity has also been verified by biochemical studies (Reichmann and Nix 1985). Another interesting finding of the present study was that properties of the contralateral muscles of the long-term stimulated side were also influenced, which makes them difficult to use as a normal control (Nix et al. 1985).

Passive electrical properties, such as membrane resistance and capacitance of single fibres in denervated muscles, have been reported to be restored to normal by intermittent activity bursts (Westgaard 1975). Mechanical latency, which depends on membrane properties, showed no difference in denervated and denervated stimulated muscle. This finding has also been reported by others (Melichna and Gutmann 1974; Fleisch et al. 1952).

Long-term stimulation has been shown to influence denervated muscle via muscle activity. The question now is whether short-term stimulation acts on the same principle. All studies that used short-term stimulation have based their interpretations on muscle weight; a few have also used morphometric methods. Studies of contractile parameters and fatigue behaviour have not been performed. Parameters for comparison with this study are, therefore, not available. This study demonstrates that short-term stimulation retards atrophy, and, parallel to this, the decline in contractile parameters is slowed. The beakdown of muscle is slowed, but this does not seem to have a specific influence on the enzyme activities.

The atrophy-retarding effect of electrical stimulation has been proven in many animal studies. The necessity for at least 20 min of daily stimulation has been stressed in these reports. Shorter stimulation regimes had no effect (Gutmann and Guttmann 1944). Both vigorous contractions and stimulation of the muscle in a stretched position are prerequisites to retard atrophy (Gutmann and Guttmann 1944; Fisher and Ramsey 1946; Fleisch et al. 1952). This demonstrates that physical parameters, especially the position of the denervated muscle, must be taken into consideration (Melichna and Gutmann 1974). Isometric stimulation, as used in this study, initiated stretch tension in the denervated muscle. Muscle stretch has previously been shown to stimulate the protein synthesis in denervated muscle (Goldspink 1978). Therefore, stretch activity would seem sufficient to explain the atrophy-retarding effect of short-term stimulation.

To achieve positive results with short-term procedures, a time factor has to be considered. Stimulation must start within days of denervation, otherwise the regime is not effective (Gutmann and Guttmann 1944). With long-term stimulation, even after longer periods of denervation, the muscle can still be influenced (Nix 1985). There was no morphological difference between the denervated and short-term stimulated muscles a few weeks after reinnervation in the denervated only and reinnervated muscle. The rate of reinnervation does not seem to be affected either (Gutmann and Guttmann 1944; Hines et al. 1945). In a recent study, short-term stimulation resulted in higher weights and tetanic forces in denervated stimulated and reinnervated muscles (Cole and Gardiner 1984). Long-term stimulation of denervated muscle had no effect on nerve regeneration, but direct stimulation of regenerating nerve increased the rate of functional recovery (Nix 1982; Nix and Hopf 1983). In partially denervated and stimulated muscles sprouting behaviour of the nerve was seen to be influenced in retarding terminal and enhancing collateral outgrowth (Brown et al. 1977; Brown and Ironton 1977). The functional significance of this observation is not yet known.

This study has shown that denervated muscle can be influenced by long-term isotonic as well as short-term isometric electrical stimulation. The effects result in either retardation of denervation-induced degradation of muscle tissue or rearrangement of enzyme composition of muscle. To study this, standardized experimental setups were necessary which involved the implantation of stimulating electrodes, a procedure only possible in animals. The result from animal work performed under specific experimental conditions are valuable for elucidating biological mechanisms. As stimulation regimes are possible in animals under conditions which are not possible in man, these experimental results cannot be used to prove the effectiveness of any form of electrical stimulation in man. It is difficult in man to achieve activation of all the fibres within a large denervated muscle bulk and to perform daily stimulation periods for different lengths of time. Technical limitations are therefore the main reason for leaving without effect the clinically used form of electrostimulation.

References

Brown MC, Ironton R (1977) Suppression of motor nerve terminal sprouting in partially denervated mouse muscle. J Physiol (Lond) 272:70–71P

Brown MC, Goodwin G, Ironton R (1977) Prevention of nerve sprouting in botulinum toxin poisoned mouse soleus muscle by direct stimulation of the muscle. J Physiol (Lond) 267:42–43P

Buller A, Eccles J, Eccles R (1960) Differentiation of fast and slow muscles in the cat hind limb. J Physiol (Lond) 150:339–370

Burke RE, Levine FE, Zajac FE, Tsairis P, Engel WK (1971) Mammalian motor units: physiological-histochemical correlation in three types of cat gastrognemius. Science 174:709–712

Cole B, Gardiner P (1984) Does electrical stimulation of denervated muscle, continued after reinnervation, influence recovery of contractile function? Exp Neurol 85:52–62

Dubowitz V, Brooke M (1973) Muscle Biopsy: A modern approach. Saunders, London

Eerbeek O, Kernell D, Verhey BA (1984) Effects of fast and slow patterns of tonic long-term stimulation on contractile properties of fast muscle in the cat. J Physiol (Lond) 352:73–90

Fischer E, Ramsey V (1946) The effect of daily stimulation of normal and denervated muscle upon their protein content and upon some of the physicochemical properties of the protein. Am J Physiol 145:583–586

Fleisch A, Estoppey J, Hofstetter J (1952) Etude expérimentale du traitment électrique des muscles paralysés. Helv Physiol Acta 10:93–109

Girlanda P, Dattola R, Vita G, Oteri G, LoPresti F, Messina C (1982) Effects of electrotherapy on denervated muscle in rabbits: an electrophysiological and morphological study. Exp Neurol 77:483–491

Goldspink D (1978) The influence of passive stretch on the growth and protein turnover of denervated extensor digitorum longus muscle. Biochem J 174:595–602

Gutmann E, Guttmann L (1944) The effect of galvanic exercise on denervated and re-innervated muscles in the rabbit. J Neurol Neurosurg Psychiatry 7:7–17

Hines H, Melville E, Wehrmacher W. (1945) The effect of electrical stimulation on neuromuscular regeneration. Am J Physiol 144:278–283

Hudlická O, Tyler K, Aitman T (1980) The effect of long-term electrical stimulation on fuel uptake and performance in fast skeletal muscle. In: Pette D (ed) Plasticity of muscle. Walter de Gruyter, Berlin, pp 401–408

Lømo T, Westgaard R, Dahl H (1974) Contractile properties of muscle: control by pattern of muscle activity in the rat. Proc R Soc Lond [Biol] 187:99–103

Lømo T, Westgaard R, Engebretsen L (1980) Different stimulation pattern affect contractile properties of denervated rat soleus muscles. In: Pette D (ed) Plasticity of muscle. Walter de Gruyter, Berlin, pp 297–309

Melichna J, Gutmann E (1974) Stimulation and immobilisation effects on contractile and histochemical properties of denervated muscle. Pflugers Arch 352:165–178

Nachmias V, Padykula H (1958) A histochemical study of normal and denervated red and white muscle of the rat. J Biophys Biochem Cytol 4:47–54

Nemeth P (1982) Electrical stimulation of denervated muscle prevents decrease in oxidative enzymes. Muscle Nerve 5:134–139

Nix WA (1982) The effect of low frequency electrical stimulation on the denervated extensor digitorum longus of the rabbit. Acta Neurol Scand 66:521–528

Nix WA (1986) Maintenance of muscle integrity following denervation. In: Dimitrijevic M, Kakulas BA, Vrbová G (eds) Recent achievements in restorative neurology. Karger, Basel (to be published)

Nix WA, Hopf HC (1983) Electrical stimulation of regenerating nerve and its effect on motor recovery. Brain Res 272:21–25

Nix WA, Heinz A, Schreiber T (1983) Elektrische Reizmuster als Faktor zur funktionellen Beeinflussung denervierter Muskulatur. In: Seitz D, Vogel P (eds) Verhandlungen der Deutschen Gesellschaft für Neurologie. Springer, Berlin Heidelberg New York, pp 823–832

Nix WA, Reichmann H, Schröder JM (1985) Influence of direct low frequency stimulation on contractile properties of denervated fast-twitch rabbit muscle. Pflugers Arch 405:141–147

Pette D, Smith M, Staudte H, Vrbová G (1973) Effects of long-term electrical stimulation on some contractile and metabolic characteristics of fast rabbit muscle. Pflugers Arch 338:257–272

Pette D, Ramirez U, Müller W, Simon R, Exner G, Hildebrandt R (1975) Influence of intermittent long term stimulation on contractile, histochemical and metabolic properties of fibre populations in fast and slow rabbit muscle. Pflugers Arch 361:1–7

Pette D, Müller W, Leisner E, Vrbová G (1976) Time dependant effects on contractile properties, fibre population, myosin light chains and enzyme metabolism in intermittent and continuously stimulated fast twitch muscle of rabbit. Pflugers Arch 364:103–112

Reichmann H, Nix WA (1985) Changes of energy metabolism, myosin light chain composition, lactate dehydrogenase isoenzyme pattern and fibre type distribution of denervated fast-twitch muscle of rabbit after low frequency stimulation. Pflugers Arch 405:244–249

Reid J (1841) On the relation between muscular contractility and the nervous system. Lond Edinb Month J Med Sci 1:320–329

Salmons S, Vrbová G (1969) The influence of activity on some contractile characteristics of mammalian fast and slow muscle. J Physiol (Lond) 201:535–549

Westgaard R (1975) Influence of activity on the passive electrical properties of denervated soleus muscle fibres in the rat. J Physiol (Lond) 251:683–697

Effects of Electrical Stimulation on Normal and Diseased Human Muscle*

O. M. Scott[1], G. Vrbová[3], S. A. Hyde[1], and V. Dubowitz[2]

Introduction

Skeletal muscle, although exhibiting a high degree of specialization, shows a remarkable ability to adapt its biochemical, physiological and ultrastructural properties in response to changes in demand. Investigations in animals have shown that it is possible to modify the properties of mammalian muscles by chronic electrical stimulation, and fast muscle fibres of both cats and rabbits have been induced to undergo a series of systematic changes which ultimately result in complete transformation to slow contracting fibres (Salmons and Vrbová 1969). There is overwhelming evidence that these changes are directly related to imposed activity and that functional and metabolic characteristics of muscle fibres depend upon the activity of the motoneuron.

Our studies have been concerned to investigate the effect of chronic low-frequency electrical stimulation on normal and diseased human muscle and were planned in three stages. The first involved establishing baseline data of muscle function in normal adults in terms of maximum voluntary contraction (MVC), the response to fatigue testing, exploring the feasibility of using prolonged low-frequency electrical stimulation in human subjects and evaluating the time course of any changes in the mechanical properties of the stimulated muscles. The second stage investigated skeletal muscle function in normal young children and a comparison was made with the data obtained from normal adults. The final stage has involved exploring the rationale of chronic low-frequency stimulation and investigating differences in the contractile properties of normal children's muscles and muscles of children with Duchenne muscular dystrophy (DMD) before proceeding to evaluate changes of muscle function and functional performance in response to prolonged stimulation.

Methods

Subjects

Three groups of subjects took part in these studies which had been approved by the Ethics Committee of the Hammersmith Hospital. Baseline date of muscle function

* This work was supported by the Medical Research Council

1 Departments of Physiotherapy and
2 Paediatrics, Hammersmith Hospital, London, W12 OHS, U.K.
3 Department of Anatomy and Embryology, Centre for Neuroscience, University College, London, WC1E 6BT, U.K.

Electrical Stimulation and Neuromuscular Disorders
Ed. by W. A. Nix and G. Vrbová

of tibialis anterior were established for 16 normal adults, 18 normal children aged from 3 to 13 years and 16 boys ranging from 5 to 12 years of age with DMD. The diagnosis was based on a clinical history of early onset and progressive muscle weakness, confirmed by muscle biopsy and exceptionally high levels of serum creatine kinase (CK).

In order to evaluate the effects of chronic low-frequency stimulation, five female adult subjects, two normal children and 14 boys with DMD undertook to stimulate their tibialis anterior muscles at a frequency of 10 Hz or less for an hour, three times daily for 6 weeks. The duration of chronic stimulation was extended to a maximum of 11 weeks in the study of children with DMD.

Selection of Muscle

The decision to use the tibialis anterior muscle was based on the accessibility of the muscle for purposes of testing and long-term stimulation, the relative insensitivity of skin in that area and therefore the anticipated high tolerance to the sensory effects of long-term stimulation. Moreover, since extensive animal studies had used this muscle, it provided for planned continuity and transference to human studies.

Chronic Low Frequency Stimulation

The subjects stimulated their tibialis anterior muscles with a small battery-operated stimulator. Stimulation was by two 4-cm-square carbon rubber electrodes placed over the motor point and the belly of the muscle; these were attached by leads to the stimulator which was worn on a belt around the waist. Good contact was ensured by electrode jelly, and the subjects were instructed to adjust the position of the two electrodes on the muscle and the output of the stimulator to give sufficient stimulation to see a visible contraction of the tibialis anterior accompanied by movement of the foot. A day-by-day chart of hours of stimulation was kept by each subject.

Muscle Function Studies

Tension recordings were made of maximum voluntary and electrically evoked contractions of the tibialis anterior muscle using a specially designed chair, a rigid foot plate and an adjustable steel bar on which strain gauges were mounted (Scott et al. 1985). Two 4-cm square carbon rubber electrodes were placed over the motor point and the belly of the muscle and a routine of testing was established to record the increments of tension in response to brief trains of stimulation at 1, 10, 20 and 40 Hz. To determine resistance to fatigue, the muscle was stimulated at 40 Hz for 250 ms every second for 5 min and the percentage decrease of tension after 3 min the fatigue index (FI) was measured. The effect of this fatigue test on the increments of tension elicited by the brief trains of stimulation was established by comparing the percentage of tension developed in response to the brief trains of stimulation at 10 and 20 Hz to that developed at 40 Hz before and after the fatigue test.

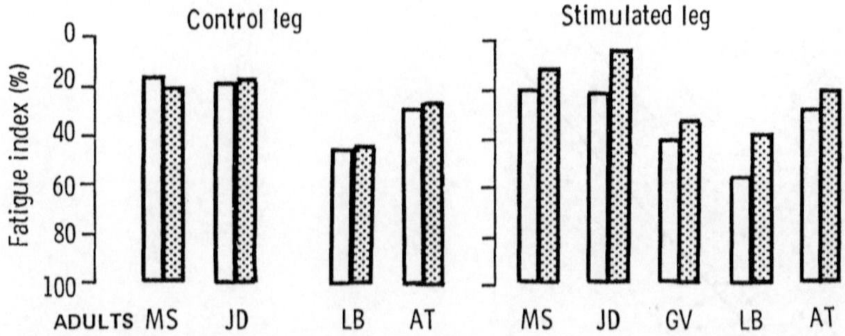

Fig. 1. Change in fatigue index following stimulation for 3 h each day at 10 Hz. □ Before stimulation; ▩ after 6 weeks stimulation

Results

Adult Subjects

Five normal adult female volunteers stimulated their tibialis anterior muscles for an hour three times daily for 6 weeks. Muscles of the contralateral legs acted as controls. Before the period of chronic stimulation, all subjects showed a characteristic decrease of tension during the fatigue test and there was no apparent difference between the muscles of either leg. Figure 1 shows that after 6 weeks of chronic stimulation there was a marked change in fatigability, and in each individual the stimulated muscles fatigued less than the unstimulated control. The ability to maintain tension was increased by 12.3% ± 5.8% whereas the overall change of the fatigue index of the control muscles during the same period was only 0.18% ± 3.5%. The difference between the fatigability of the control and stimulated muscles was highly significant ($P<0.01$); thus, chronic low-frequency stimulation enhanced the ability of the muscles to maintain tension.

There was no corresponding change in the MVC during the same period, and there was no apparent difference in the percentage of tension developed at 10 Hz and 20 Hz before and after the fatigue test was assessed in the control or chronically stimulated muscles. This suggests that while chronic stimulation increased the fatigue resistance of the muscle after 6 weeks of 3 h stimulation daily, it did not have an appreciable effect on the contractile properties.

Normal Children

Figure 2 shows that there was a linear relationship and a high correlation of 0.92 when the MVC exerted by the anterior tibial muscles of both legs of 18 normal children was plotted against age.

Table 1 shows that about 22% of the MVC was activated on stimulation at 40 Hz. Unlike adults, the effect of fatigue testing at 40 Hz for 5 minutes resulted in little or no decrease of the initial tension developed by the muscle and following the fatigue

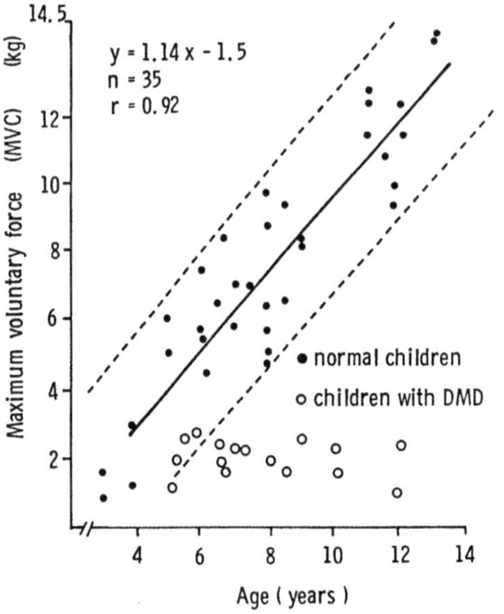

Fig. 2. Relationships of maximum voluntary contraction *(MVC)* of dorsiflexors of ankle of 16 children with Duchenne muscular dystrophy to age. A comparison is made with the same relationship between strength and age in normal children; the regression line and 95% confidence limits are shown

Table 1. Fatigue Test. Comparison of mean values ± SD of MVC, fatigue indices and ratios of 10/40 and 20/40 Hz before and after fatigue testing of right legs of 18 normal children and 16 children with DMD

	Normal children ($n = 18$)		DMD children ($n = 16$)	
	Before	After	Before	After
EEC[a] kg	1.8 ± 1.2	1.8 ± 1.1	0.45 ± 0.18	0.41 ± 0.12
% MVC	22.1 ± 9.3	20.1 ± 10.1	28.9 ± 11.0	26.0 ± 11.2
Fatigue index (FI) %	−1.5 ± 19.1		5.5 ± 8.1	
Tension at				
10 Hz[b]	19.3 ± 8.9	27.2 ± 6.6	24.0 ± 9.7	21.0 ± 11.9
20 Hz[b]	56.9 ± 11.9	62.0 ± 9.9	55.6 ± 10.3	53.6 ± 11.9

[a] EEC, electrically elicited contraction at 40 Hz ± SD
[b] Tension expressed at % of tension developed at 40 Hz

test, there was no change of tension on restimulation at 40 Hz. There was, however, a significant increase in the proportion of tension developed on stimulation at 10 Hz following completion of the fatigue test and a similar but smaller and more variable increase of tension on restimulation at 20 Hz.

There was no apparent change in the MVC of the two normal children, aged 9 and 11 years respectively, following 6 weeks of three hours daily of low-frequency stimulation and no change was demonstrated in their high resistance to fatigue or in the percentages of tension developed in response to the selected frequencies of stimulation following completion of the period of stimulation.

Children with Duchenne Muscular Dystrophy

The muscle strength of children with DMD does not increase with age. Figure 2 shows the MVC exerted by the anterior tibial muscles of the stronger leg of the 16 children compared with the MVC exerted by the same muscle group in 18 normal children. In younger DMD children, it can be seen that the MVC falls within the range of the lower limits of normal strength.

Table 1 compares the electrically elicited responses of the right tibialis anterior muscle of 16 children with DMD and those of 18 normal children. It can be seen that the results are comparable, about 26% of the MVC was activated by electrical stimulation at 40 Hz; as in normal children's muscles a minimal loss of tension was sustained in response to prolonged stimulation for 5 minutes at this frequency, and no change of tension was observed on restimulation at 40 Hz following completion of the fatigue test. However, in the muscles of children with DMD, there was no post-fatigue potentiation and no increase of force was recorded on restimulation at 10 or 20 Hz.

Eight boys with DMD took part in an initial feasibility study to investigate the effects of chronic low-frequency stimulation to identify any practical problems which might arise, to evaluate the chosen parameters of stimulation and to ascertain if any changes occurred in the mechanical properties of the stimulated muscles. As a result of this study, modifications were made both in the selection of children and the parameters of chronic low-frequency stimulation. The pattern of chronic stimulation was changed from continuous to intermittent stimulation (cycle 1.5 s on 1.5 s off) and children unable to climb stairs or with fixed equinus deformities greater than 20° loss of dorsiflexion were excluded from the study.

Six boys took part in the next stage of the study. All the boys sustained excellent records of compliance with the planned programme of stimulation. The mean age of these boys was 7.2 ± 1.8 years and the mean period of stimulation was 8.7 ± 1.4 weeks. Table 2 shows that there was a small but significant increase ($P < 0.05$) of

Table 2. Maximum voluntary strength (MVC) of 6 boys with Duchenne muscular dystrophy before and after intermittent chronic low-frequency stimulation (6–8 Hz)

Subject	Age (years)	Weeks of stimulation	Control leg		Stimulated leg		Difference	
			Before	After	Before	After	Control	Stimulated
1	10.0	10	1.8	1.3	1.7	2.6	−0.5	+0.9
2	8.5	9	1.7	1.8	0.9	1.6	+0.1	+0.7
3	7.2	10	1.5	1.9	2.0	1.6	+0.4	−0.4
4	6.7	7	1.9	1.9	1.7	2.4	0	+0.7
5	5.3	9	1.7	1.8	2.2	2.6	+0.1	+0.4
6	5.5	7	2.0	2.6	1.7	3.0	0.6	+1.3
Mean	7.2	8.7	1.8	1.9	1.7	2.3	0.1	0.6
± SD	1.8	1.4	0.2	0.4	0.4	0.6	0.4	0.6

Before, mean value of 1st and 2nd assessment
After, mean value on completion of stimulation and 1 month later

0.6 kg ± 0.6 of the strength of the chronically stimulated muscles compared with a minimal change of 0.1 kg ± 0.4 of the control muscles. There was no change in the fatigue indices after chronic low-frequency stimulation, nor did analysis of the tensions developed in response to brief trains of stimulation at 10 and 20 Hz before and after fatigue, expressed as a percentage of the tension evoked at 40 Hz, show any apparent change in these ratios following prolonged low-frequency stimulation.

Discussion

These studies have established the feasibility of subjecting the muscles of human subjects to prolonged low-frequency electrical stimulation. Although there was a need for clear and precise instructions and a reliable support service for minor repairs to the stimulators, it was realistic to consider the use of low-frequency stimulators on an outpatient home-care basis.

Investigations in rats and rabbits have shown that prolonged stimulation of fast skeletal muscles causes them to become fatigue resistant (Hudlická et al. 1977), and the present study shows that this change also occurs in the tibialis anterior muscles of normal adult subjects. An increase in the MVC was not anticipated, only small increases of tetanic tension had been observed following chronic low-frequency stimulation (Pette et al. 1973) and experience of the effect of exercise in human subjects, for review see Holloszy and Booth (1976), together with the results of chronic stimulation in animals suggest that the adaption that could be expected would be an increased capacity of the muscle for aerobic metabolism and an increase of endurance. It is possible that the total time that the muscles were stimulated (3 h each day for 6 weeks) was insufficient to complete the changes of the contractile properties or to result in transformation in muscle fibre type composition.

The finding that there was no decrease of the initial tension in young children's muscle in response to the fatigue test was unexpected and revealed a difference in mechanical performance between normal mature adult muscle and young children's muscles. Further studies have shown that minimal changes in the time course of contraction during the 5-min test or on restimulation at 40 Hz after completion of the test (Scott et al. 1985). The explanation for the lack of fatigue may be accounted for by the smaller diameters of children's muscle fibres and the probability that the more efficient supply of oxygen makes the muscles more resistant to fatigue. Roe and his colleagues (1967) also found that muscles of children with DMD were very difficult to fatigue and observed that normal children showed the same high resistance to fatigue. The differences in post-tetanic potentiation found between normal children's muscles and those of children with DMD before and after the fatigue test may indicate that the mechanism by which the onset of fatigue is prevented differs in muscles of Duchenne children from that of normal children.

Chronic low-frequency stimulation in the dystrophic mouse muscle was shown to induce enzyme and membrane properties characteristic of adult fast muscle (Dangain and Vrbová 1982) and has also been shown to reduce the rate of deterioration in dystrophic mice and chickens (Reichmann et al. 1981; Barnard et al. 1984). Improvement in function and an increase of muscle fibres together with raised oxidative levels, higher tensions and reduced time courses of contraction in dystrophic mouse muscle have been reported (Luthert et al. 1980; Vrbová and Ward 1981).

The change of the pattern of stimulation in association with the selection of subjects at earlier stages of the disease may account for the increase of strength found in the second study of the effect of chronic low-frequency stimulation on DMD muscles.

Summary

The results of our investigations have shown that the properties of human muscles were changed in response to superimposed electrical activity. The method of treatment was found to be acceptable and it was possible to evaluate both the increase in resistance to fatigue, which occurred in normal adult tibialis anterior muscle in response to prolonged chronic low-frequency electrical stimulation, and the significant increase in MVC in the same muscle of young children with DMD in response to intermittent chronic stimulation at 6–8 Hz when compared with the tension exerted by the control muscles of the other leg.

Acknowledgements. We are grateful to Biomedical Research Limited for donating some stimulators.

References

Barnard EA, Barnard P, Jarvis JC, Lai J (1984) Low frequency stimulation in vivo of chick fast-twitch muscle. J Physiol (Lond) 351:37p

Dangain J, Vrbová G (1982) Effects of low frequency stimulation on the passive membrane properties of muscle fibres from dystrophic mice. In: Fifth international congress on neuromuscular diseases, Marseilles (abstract)

Holloszy JO, Booth FW (1976) Biochemical adaptions to endurance exercise in muscle. Am Rev Physiol 38:273–291

Hudlická O, Brown MD, Cotter M, Smith ME, Vrbová G (1977) The effect of long-term stimulation of fast muscle on their blood flow, metabolism and ability to withstand fatigue. Pflugers Arch 369:141–149

Luthert P, Vrbová G, Ward KM (1980) Effects of slow frequency electrical stimulation on muscles of dystrophic mice. J Neurol Neurosurg Psychiatry 43:803–809

Pette D, Smith ME, Staudte HW, Vrbová G (1973) Effects of long-term stimulation on some contractile and metabolic characteristics of fast rabbit muscle. Pflugers Arch 338:257–272

Reichmann H, Pette D, Vrbová G (1981) Effects of low frequency electrical stimulation on enzyme and isoenzyme patterns of dystrophic mouse. FEBS Lett 128:55–58

Roe RD, Yamaji K, Sandow A (1967) Contractile responses of dystrophic muscles of mouse and man. In: Milhorat AT (ed) Exploratory concepts in muscular dystrophy and related disorders. Exerpta Medica, Amsterdam, pp 299–304

Salmons S, Vrbová G (1969) The influence of activity on some contractile characteristics of mammalian fast and slow muscles. J Physiol (Lond) 201:535–549

Scott OM, Vrbová G, Hyde SA, Dubowitz V (1985) Effects of chronic low frequency electrical stimulation on normal human tibialis anterior muscle. J Neurol Neurosurg Psychiatry 48:774–781

Vrbová G, Ward K (1981) Observations on the effects of low frequency electrical stimulation on fast muscles of dystrophic mice. J Neurol Neurosurg Psychiatry 44:1002–1006

Treatment of Idiopathic Scoliosis with Daily Short-Term Electrostimulation

O. Schmitt[1]

Introduction

Bayer (1957) first reported on electrostimulation in idiopathic scoliosis. His electromyographic investigations showed increased activity in paravertebral muscles at the convexity of scoliotic curves. He thus concluded that a weakness of the contralateral muscles was the cause for the development of the deformity and therefore stimulated at the concave side. Later investigations (Brussatis 1962; Schmitt 1981) showed that this conception of the etiology of idiopathic scoliosis was wrong, and furthermore, that the therapeutic dissection of the rami dorsales of spinal nerves (Riddle and Roaf 1955) to weaken the erector spinae muscle at the convexity must have disastrous consequences.

Some years ago new activities began in this field, when in animal experiments scoliotic deformities produced by paravertebral muscle stimulation could be corrected by applying electrostimulation on the contralateral side and consequently at the convexity of scoliosis (Monticelli et al. 1975; Olsen et al. 1975, 1977).

Later, several electrostimulation methods were developed with an implanted system (Bobechko 1974) as well as with skin electrodes (Axelgaard et al. 1978). With the implanted system only erector spinae muscle is stimulated. Surface electrodes are placed on lateral muscle groups, where inter alia intercostal muscles are also reached from the electrical stimulation field to produce a better correction of the deformity than with stimulation of erector spinae muscle alone. But both muscle groups exert a stabilising function on the spine and therefore must be taken into consideration when performing electrostimulation to prevent increase of spinal deformity. Both methods described use low-frequency pulse series (about 30 Hz) consisting of short pulses (up to 200 µs). To obtain a therapeutic effect, long-term stimulation methods must be performed during the night over a period of 7–10 h thus causing many problems in respect to skin reactions and tolerable stimulation strength. In addition, available stimulators do not exactly provide the desired rectangular pulse form which is very important for the stimulation result.

We therefore developed another device, which permits simultaneous stimulation of both the paravertebral muscles and the intercostal muscles. For this purpose we used sufficiently strong constant current rectangular pulses of 1 ms duration with high frequency (100 Hz) to obtain in addition a muscular training effect. This method permits a stimulation time of only 20 min a day.

1 Orthopaedic University Hospital, 6650 Homburg/Saar, F.R.G.

Electrical Stimulation and Neuromuscular Disorders
Ed. by W. A. Nix and G. Vrbová

General Aspects of the Clinical Application of Electrostimulation in Idiopathic Scoliosis

The aim of electrostimulation is to restore the morphology and/or function of muscles in order to normalize pathologically changed stability and movement of the affected skeletal region. The earlier the clinical development is recognized and therapy is applied, the better is the influence on reversible morphological and/or functional changes.

The identification of muscles suitable for electrostimulation must take biomechanical facts as well as electromyographic and histological examinations into consideration.

Biomechanical considerations are necessary to identify those muscles responsible for, or afflicted by, the pathologically alterated stability or motion of the affected skeletal region. Electromyographic investigations have to be performed in order to examine the activity of these muscles in function. With histological examinations the extent of morphological and histochemically seizeable alterations significant for the function of muscle (fibre diameter and type constellation) can be characterized.

Clinical Development of Idiopathic Scoliosis

Many investigations have been performed on the clinical appearance of idiopathic scoliosis on the genetic determination of the disease, prevailing in females (Wynne-Davis 1973; MacEwen and Cowell 1970; Brooks et al. 1973; Robin and Cohen 1975). It could be shown that growth and hormonal factors in puberty have an important influence on the progression of deformities (Duval-Beaupere 1971; Willner 1972).

Our own investigations additionally showed, that various forms could be classified in slight (A), middle (B) and heavy (C) scoliosis by measuring the angle and extensibility of the deformity with respect to age at the beginning of treatment (Schmitt 1981).

With equal sex distribution (0.7:1) patients from group A developed slight deformities of about 10 degrees before the age of 10 years (after Lippmann and Cobb). Only after the age of 10 is there a slight prevalance of females (2.8:1). Patients in group B are mainly females (11:1). At the age of about 12 years they suddenly develop curves of about 30 degrees. The extensibility decreases with further growth. This decrease of extensibility has to be considered as a sign of structural stabilization. Such curves are obviously cured during treatment. Patients of group C (also dominantly females 5:1) have at the age of about 10 an earlier developed, and at this time already structurally stabilized, curve of about 30 degrees. Later, an occurring instability elucidated by increasing extensibility once again causes a loosening of the temporarily stabilized and earlier developed curves. In these cases operative treatment becomes necessary at a later date in order to prevent secondary complications.

Looking at the external form of scoliosis it can be seen that patients from group B and C show a significant prevalance of right convexity in the thoracal region. The number of segments increases as the deformity progresses.

Because the etiology of the disease is unknown and a causative treatment is therefore not possible, as much data as possible has to be collected so that an answer to the future behaviour of the individual curve can be provided. These known facts have to be taken into consideration when determining when to begin electrostimulation treatment.

Identification of Muscles

Biomechanical considerations show that under physiological conditions the stability of the spine is generally guaranteed by the connective tissue, especially the discs, muscles and skeletal structures. Static stability is mainly provided by the ribs, stabilising rotational movement as well as side bending forces supported by inter-

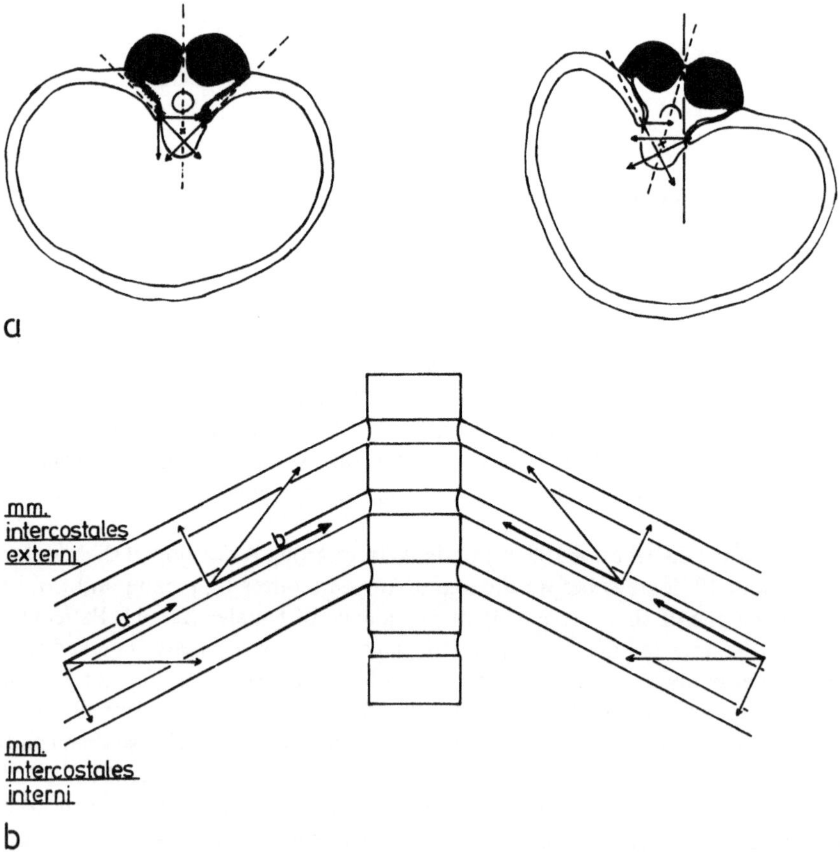

Fig. 1a, b. The rib levers act together with the m. erector spinae as excellent rotational stabilizators in normal spine (**a** *left*). With increasing scoliotic deformity the deforming vector at the concave side increases whereas the stabilizing vector at the convexity decreases (**a** *right*). Thus the spine comes into a disequilibrium with increasing deformity in rotational and side-bending stabilization. The electrostimulation of m. erector spinae and m. intercostales counteracts against the rotational and the increasing side-bending deformation (**b**)

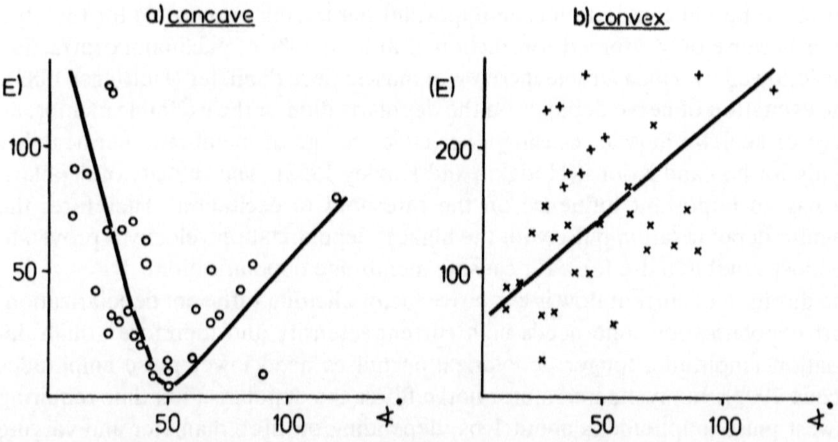

Fig. 2a, b. With the increase of scoliotic deformity, the rest activity of intercostal muscles at the convex side increases (**b**) whereas the activity of the same muscle group at the concave side decreases, followed by an increase of activities in heavy curves (**a**)

costal muscles giving them a dynamic adaptability. Paravertebral muscles of the same side have in this sence a synergistic function stabilizing both movements (Fig. 1).

Electromyographic investigations have shown that under normal resting conditions the intercostal muscles are symmetrically activated. But obviously there are reflectory interactions between the activities of the upper extremities to stabilize the contralateral side of the thoraxic spine if one arm is carrying a load. Lateralization (prevailing of right hand activities) may be one cause of prevailing and progression tendency of right convexities in the thoraxic spine. In scoliotic spine intercostal muscles as well as paravertebral muscles show an increased activity at the convexity to act against an increase of deformity (Fig. 2).

Histological and histochemical examinations show fibre atrophy and a slight increase of fat content, especially in severe deformities. The normal fibre type constellation consisting of a significant prevailing of muscles with the histochemical characteristics of slow (aerobic) types is disturbed to the disadvantage of twitch fibres (anaerobic) significantly reducing their percentage from about 37% to 25%. These changes have to be considered as the morphological and histochemical expression of a functional and metabolic disturbance of muscles (Schmitt 1981, 1985).

Stimulation Parameters

The nerve function on muscles is twofold: the motor function transmitting the excitation to the muscle membrane to produce muscle contraction and the trophic function maintaining ability and force of muscle contraction and influencing the contraction velocity (Schmidt and Stefani 1977; Schmidt 1980).

Artificial stimulation of nondenervated muscle enables the type as well as the diameter of muscle fibres to be influenced (Golisch et al. 1970; Pette et al. 1972, 1973).

The force of muscle contraction is an important parameter responsible for the fibre diameter because only a forced contraction of at least 50% of maximum contraction force is followed by a measurable increase of muscle fibre diameter (Hettinger 1983).

The excitation of nerve depends on the depolarisation of the excitable membrane of nerve or skeletal muscle, causing a selective change of membrane permeability especially for Na- and K-ions (Hodgkin and Huxley 1952). The velocity of depolarization has an important influence on the threshold to excitation. Therefore, the rectangular depolarisation pulse with the highest depolarization velocity is proved to be the most suitable pulse form for causing membrane depolarisation.

The duration of current flow is a decisive factor eliciting sufficient depolarization. A short depolarisation time needs high current intensity and therefore a high depolarisation amplitude; longer depolarization pulses need lower pulse amplitudes (Lapicque 1909). In myelinated motor nerve fibres the depolarisation time requiring the lowest pulse amplitude is about 1 ms, depending on fibre diameter and varying from one node to the other in the range of about 50% (Stämpfli 1971).

The threshold to excitation of the motor nerve is lower than in muscle membrane. Thus, artificial muscle stimulation, especially with surface electrodes, will be more effective at stimulating motor nerves than muscle membranes. The large neural fibres supplying the fast motor units have a lower threshold than the small fibres supplying the slow motor units. In addition, the muscle anatomy is such that the fast, fatigable muscle fibres tend to be located superficially to the slow, more fatigue-resistant fibres (Mortimer 1981).

Using surface electrodes an electric stimulation field is applied over structures for depolarization. The current density of this field has to be choosen so that the amount of ion movement is adequate for the depolarization of the membrane areas to be excited. This depends on the size and positioning of the electrodes. Small closely spaced electrodes make the effective area of stimulation rather superficial, whereas larger electrodes spaced further apart facilitate the stimulation of deeper tissue. The actual current density at any particular point within the tissue will vary depending on tissue impedance. Bone and adipose tissue, which are of relatively high impedance, are lowering the current density at the desired region of stimulation. In addition, with increasing distance from the electrodes the increasing tissue impedance and capacity causes a deformation of the applied depolarising pulse, resulting in a decrease of amplitude and depolarization velocity.

The results of electromyographic and histological investigations must be taken into consideration when choosing suitable stimulation parameters for restoring reversible pathological changes of muscles in idiopathic scoliosis. This means removing atrophy and restoring metabolic and functional conditions for normal fibre type constellation, followed by an increase of fibres with anaerobic metabolism (twitch fibres).

To remove fibre atrophy electrostimulation has to provoke strong enough muscle contractions for redressing and growth control of scoliotic spine. The regeneration of twitch fibres is striven for, using high-frequency pulse series. In order to stimulate paravertebral muscles as well as intercostal muscles simultaneously, depending on their physiological synergistic function, we have to apply a strong electrical field consisting of long rectangular single-pulse series to produce a sufficient depolarisation with minimal current.

We realized this in a three-channel electronic arrangement (Scolimax) delivering constant current rectangular pulses of 1-ms duration with increasing and decreasing pulse series reaching a plateau phase with a maximum of about 80 mA in amplitude of about 1-s duration.

Stimulation Method

With regard to the clinical application of electrostimulation, the indication of therapy must initially be decided. This depends on the history of scoliosis, the actual state of the deformation (extensibility, number of segments, localization and direction of convexity) and the special data of the individual patient (Sex, puberty, bone age). With the help of these data it must then be decided in each individual case whether electrostimulation is already indicated, or whether the deformity is so severe that a brace must be prescribed as a pretreatment for operative stabilization. The localization of electrodes should be determined after making an X-ray. They are placed in the midline of paravertebral muscle at the apex of scoliosis. In cases with lumbar curves, two electrodes are additionally placed on the oblique abdominal muscles at the concavity to obtain a further correction over traction on fascia lumbodorsalis. To improve the correction force of the paravertebral muscle, lumbar lordosis is corrected by a roll placed under the abdomen in prone position. The current has to be high enough so that strong contraction of intercostal muscles can be felt by the palpating finger and both paravertebral and oblique abdomini muscles show strong contractions. The duration of stimulation is 20 min per day.

Using this method we treated 52 patients and were able to consequently control curve development in 40 cases (6 males, 34 females) beginning 1 year before treatment over the following 5 years to about 2.5 years after the end of treatment. The average age was 13.7 years. The form of scoliosis consisted in 36 cases of a thoracic scoliosis with right convexity. In 4 cases there was a S-shaped scoliosis with right thoracal convexity. The Risser signs were 0 = 20%, I = 25%, II = 48%, III = 7%.

Results of Treatment

The correction effect depended on the degree of the deformity and the extent of structural changes. Slight curves with a short history were easier to correct than heavy curves with structural fixation (Fig. 3).

Regarding the history of scoliosis, there was an increase of curvatures of on average 31% before the beginning of treatment. After 1 year of stimulation there was a decrease of 26.5% compared with the initial value. In the following period there was no change of mean angles (Fig. 4). Obviously, most scoliotic deformities were stabilized showing on average, even 2.5 years after the end of treatment, no significant change of deformities. In detail, 44% of all patients showed a reduction of scoliotic angles of more than 5 degrees. 50% were unchanged, 6% worsened (Fig. 5).

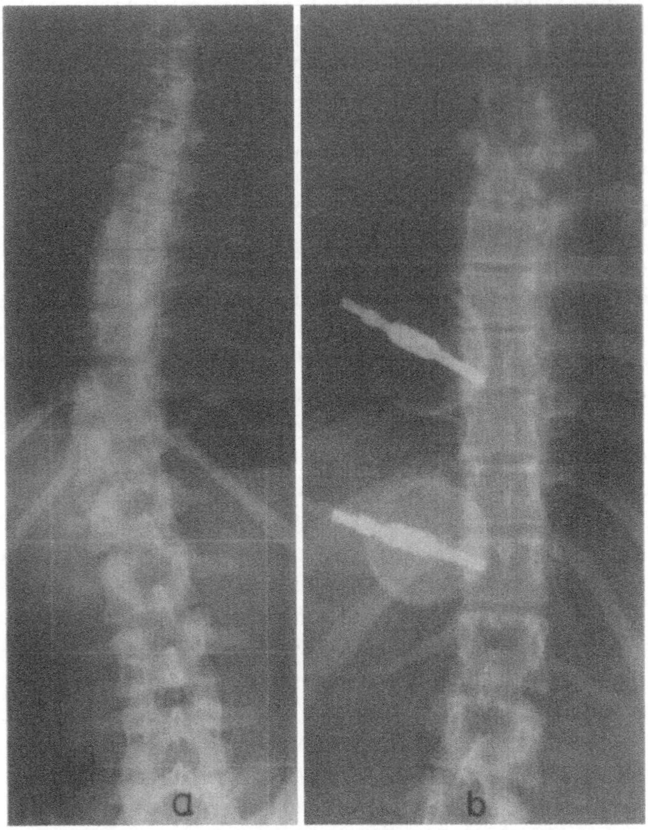

Fig. 3a, b. This X-ray shows the excellent redressing effect during stimulation to the side-bending (**a** from 30 degress to **b** almost 0 degrees) and rotational deformity

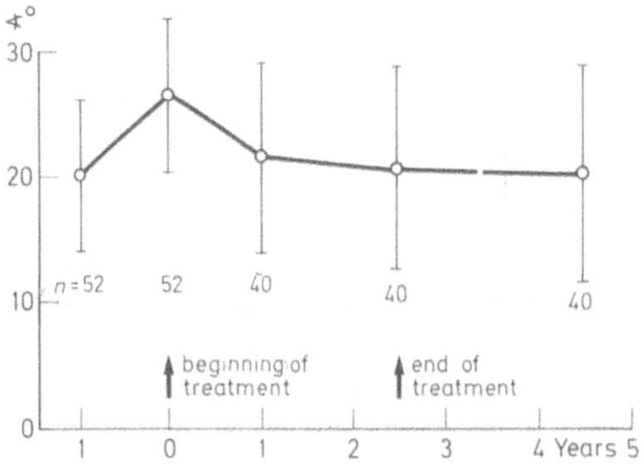

Fig. 4. After the beginning of treatment with daily short-term stimulation, the increasing tendency of all curves is stopped followed by a decrease of the mean angles in the first year of treatment. There was no change of the mean value of all treated curves to the end of treatment after 2.5 years of stimulation. The control measurement about 2.7 years after the end of treatment showed the same mean value

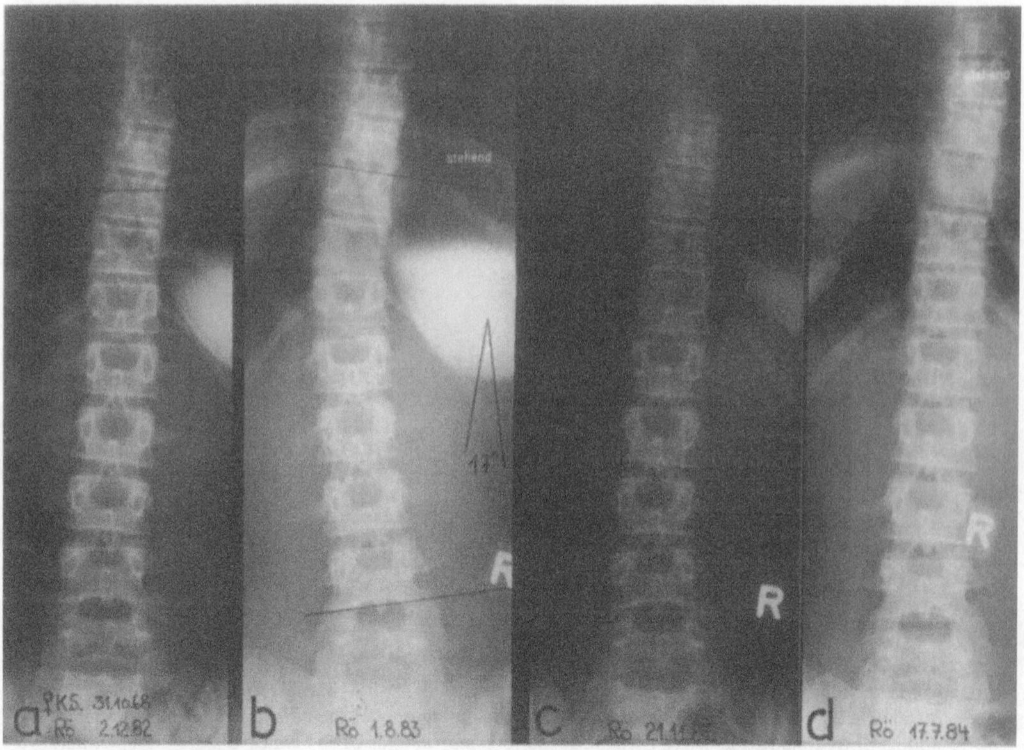

Fig. 5a–d. Example of a good treatment result of a 14-year-old girl with a developing thoracolumbar curve of 17 degrees (**a, b**). Three months after beginning of treatment the deformity was completely removed (**c**). Eight months later there was no significant change of the spine shape (**d**)

The electromyographic control of stimulated paravertebral muscle with body lifting in prone position showed a significant decrease of activity reduced after 10 months of treatment of half of the initial value (Fig. 6). Repeatedly performed measurements showed that at the beginning of treatment the subsequent activity values increased as a sign of muscle fatigue. This increase of muscle activity disappeared during treatment. Both effects were reversible once more showing the initial values 4 months after the end of the treatment. This electromyographically measurable effect was only to be observed in patients treated with short-term stimulation performed during the day (Fig. 7).

Comparison with Other Stimulation Methods Performed at Night

Compared with the results of lateral surface stimulation (arrest of progression or curve reduction in 84%) (Axelgaard et al. 1978; Altekruse and Heine 1985) the

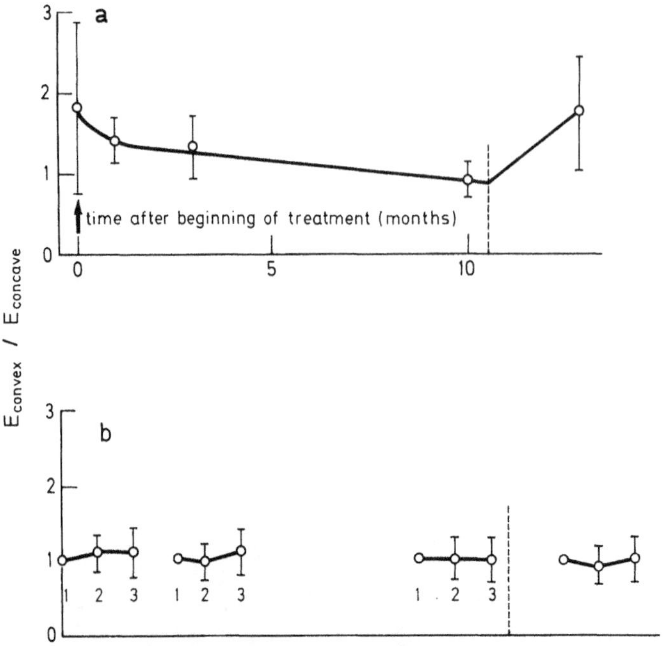

Fig. 6a, b. The electromyographic control of stimulated paravertebral muscle with body lifting in a prone position. Before the beginning of treatment **a** with daily short-term stimulation, the activity of this muscle was 1.8 higher than the activity of the same muscle of the concave side. After about 10 months of treatment this activity was reduced to same value as of the concave side. **b** Repeatedly performed measurements showed that at the beginning of treatment the subsequent activity values increased as a sign of muscle fatigue. This increase of muscle activity disappeared during treatment. Both effects were reversible again showing initial values 4 months after the end of the treatment

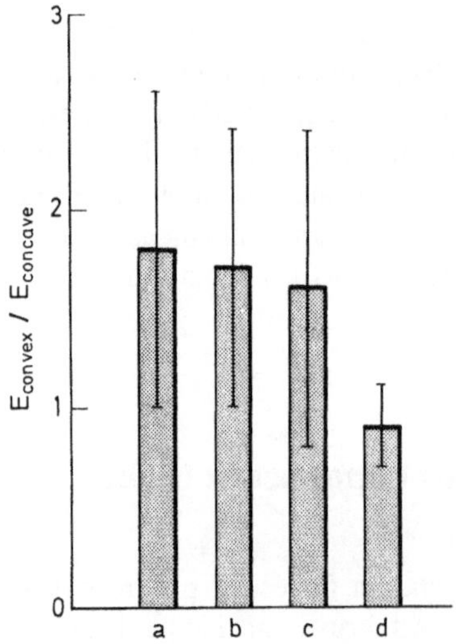

Fig. 7. Electric muscle activity of m. erector spinae with body lifting in prone position at the level of the scoliotic deformity *(a)*. Eleven months after stimulation with skin electrodes during the night *(b)* or with implanted electrodes *(c)* there was no significant change from the mean value recorded at the beginning of treatment. After the same time patients treated daily with short-term stimulation showed a significant decrease of the initial value *(d)*

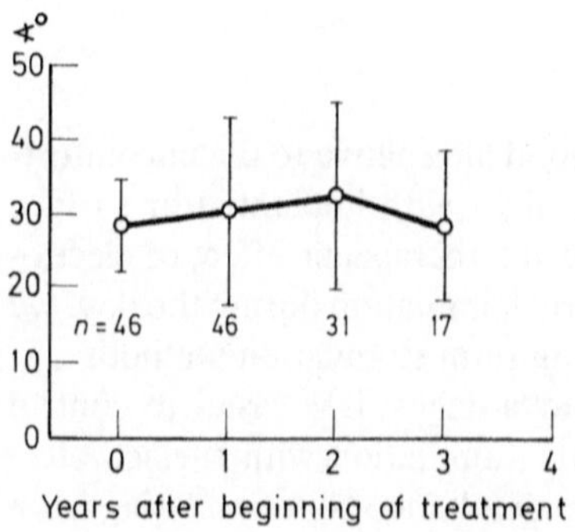

Fig. 8. Early results of treatment with implanted electrodes in idiopathic scoliosis. The stimulated muscle was m. erector spinae (66% thoracal, 17% thoracolumbar, 17% lumbar curves). The mean age at the beginning of treatment was 13.3 years (±4.3). The Risser signs were distributed as follows: 0 and 1, 76%; 2, 24%

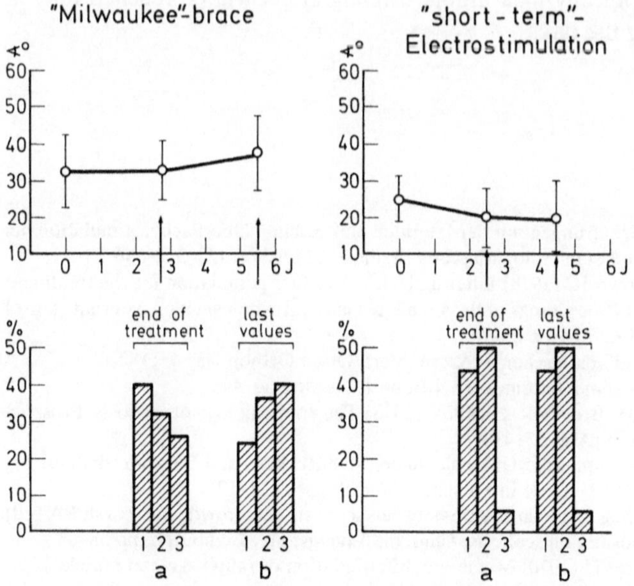

Fig. 9. The results of daily short-term stimulation (28 thoracal, 3 s-shaped scoliosis) compared with results of treatment with a Milwaukee brace (35 thoracal, 8 s-shaped scoliosis) *(above)*. The percentage of various results (*1,* better; *2,* unchanged; *3,* worsened) was examined at the end of treatment *(a)* with both methods and about 2.7 or 2 years after the end of treatment *(b)* *(below)*

results of short-term stimulation were similar. In our casuistic, the percentage of progressed curves was even lower.

Our own results with implanted electrodes show a slight reduction of the mean values of all curves over the first years after the beginning of treatment (Fig. 8).

Compared with the results of Milwaukee-brace treatment, the patients treated with short-term stimulation showed a better curve development, especially with regard to the long-term results after the end of treatment. At this time, their mean scoliotic angles were nearly constant, whereas those patients treated with a brace showed on average a slight increase of deformities (Fig. 9).

Conclusions

Electrostimulation can therefore be regarded as a good alternative to the uncomfortable brace treatment. The stimulation during the night with implanted or surface electrodes limits the compatibility and therefore also the therapeutic effect of electrostimulation. With the described method of short-term stimulation during the day, we could avoid the disadvantages of nightly applied long-term stimulation methods.

The described method therefore offers many advantages: it is easier to control and causes no skin problems in contrast to nightly stimulation with surface electrodes. The stimulation parameters are suitable for simultaneously stimulating from one unique stimulation point those muscles stabilizing scoliotic spine. Stronger muscle contractions which are more favourable for the desired training effect are tolerated. The electromyographically measurable training effect will be reached only in patients stimulated during the day.

References

Altekruse F, Heine J (1985) Erfahrungen mit der lateralen elektrischen Oberflächenstimulation bei der Behandlung der progredienten idiopathischen Skoliose. Z Orthop 123:338–346

Axelgaard J, McNeal DR, Brown JC (1978) Lateral electrical surface stimulation for the treatment of progressive scoliosis. In: Proceedings of the sixth international symposium on external control of human extremities. Dubrovnik, pp 63–70

Bayer H (1957) Ätiologie der idiopathischen Skoliose. Verh Dtsch Orthop Ges 45:182

Bobechko WP (1974) Scoliosis spinal pacemakers. J Bone Joint Surg 56:442

Brooks L, Gerberg E, Mazur H, Brooks R, Nickel V (1973) The epidemiology of scoliosis. Prospective study. J Bone Joint Surg [Am] 55:436

Brussatis F (1962) Elektromyographische Untersuchungen der Rücken- und Bauchmuskulatur bei idiopathischen Skoliosen. Wirbelsäule in Forschung und Praxis 24:1–125

Duval-Beaupere G (1971) Pathogenic relationship between scoliosis and growth. In: Zorab PA (ed) Proceedings of third symposium on scoliosis. Churchill Livingstone, Edinburgh, pp 58–64

Golisch G, Pette D, Pichelmaier H (1970) Metabolic differentiation of rabbit skeletal muscle as induced by specific innervation. Eur J Biochem 16:110–116

Hettinger T (1983) Isometrisches Muskeltraining. Thieme, Stuttgart

Hodgkin AL, Huxley AF (1952) Currents carried by sodium and potassium ions through the membrane of the giant axon of loligo. J Physiol 116:449–472

Lapicque (1971) cited in Stämpfli (1971)

MacEwen GD, Cowell HR (1970) Familial incidence of idiopathic scoliosis and its implications in patient treatment. J Bone Joint Surg [Am] 52:405

Monticelli G, Ascani E, Salsano V, Salsano A (1975) Experimental scoliosis induced by prolonged minimal electrical stimulation of the paravertebral muscles. Ital J Orthop Traumatol 1:1

Mortimer JT (1981) Motor prostheses. In: The handbook of physiology vol, III. The nervous system. Am Physiol Soc, Bethesda

Olsen GA, Rosen H, Stole S, Brown G (1975) The use of muscle stimulation for inducing scoliotic curves – a preliminary report. Clin Orthop 113:198

Olsen GA, Rosen H, Hohn RB, Slocum B (1977) Electrical muscle stimulation as a means of correction induced canine scoliotic curves. Clin Orthop 125:227–235

Pette D, Staudte HE, Vrbová G (1972) Physiological and biochemical changes induced by long term stimulation of fast muscle. Naturwissenschaften 10:469–470

Pette D, Smith MS, Staudte HE, Vrbová G (1973) Effects of long term electrical stimulation on some contractile and metabolic characteristics of fast rabbit muscles. Pflugers Arch 338:257–272

Riddle AVFV, Roaf R (1955) Muscle imbalance in the causation of scoliosis. Lancet 1:1245–1247
Robin CG, Cohen T (1975) Familial scoliosis. J Bone Joint Surg [Br] 57:146–147
Schmidt H (1980) Neural control of contractile and membrane properties in slow muscle fibres of the frog. In: Pette D (ed) Plasticity of muscle. Konstanz. Walter de Gruyter, Berlin, pp 311–324
Schmidt H, Stefani E (1977) Action potentials in slow muscle fibres of the frog during regeneration of motor nerves. J Physiol (Lond) 270:507–517
Schmitt O (1981) Zur Pathogenese der idiopathischen Thoracalskoliose und ihrer Frühbehandlung durch Elektrostimulation. Habilitationsschrift, Saarland University, Saarbrücken
Schmitt O (1985) Skoliosefrühbehandlung durch Elektrostimulation. Otte, Schlegel (eds) Bücherei des Orthopäden, vol 45. Enke, Stuttgart
Stämpfli R (1971) Physiologie des peripheren Nerven. In: von Gauer OH, Kramer K, Jung R (eds) Physiologie des Menschen, vol 10: Allgemeine Neurophysiologie. Urban and Schwarzenberg, München
Willner S (1972) Factors contributing to structural scoliosis. Thesis, University of Lund

Subject Index

GPSR Compliance

The European Union's (EU) General Product Safety Regulation (GPSR) is a set of rules that requires consumer products to be safe and our obligations to ensure this.

If you have any concerns about our products, you can contact us on ProductSafety@springernature.com

In case Publisher is established outside the EU, the EU authorized representative is:

Springer Nature Customer Service Center GmbH
Europaplatz 3
69115 Heidelberg, Germany

Batch number: 10761697

Printed by Printforce, the Netherlands